INTERFERON 3

1981

Academic Press

Interferon 1981

Interferon 1981

Volume 3

ION GRESSER
Editor-in-chief

1981

ACADEMIC PRESS

London New York Toronto Sydney San Francisco

A Subsidiary of Harcourt Brace Jovanovich, Publishers

ACADEMIC PRESS INC. (LONDON) LTD.
24/28 Oval Road,
London NW1

United States Edition published by
ACADEMIC PRESS INC.
111 Fifth Avenue
New York, New York 10003

British Library Cataloguing in Publication Data

Interferon. — Vol. 3 (1981)
1. Interferons
616.07'9 QR187.5

ISBN 0-12-302252-5

LCCCN 79-41412

Phototypeset by Dobbie Typesetting Service, Plymouth, Devon
and printed by T. J. Press (Padstow) Ltd., Cornwall

Contributors

L. B. Epstein, *Cancer Research Institute and Department of Pediatrics, University of California, San Francisco, California 94143, USA*

P. Lengyel, *Department of Molecular Biophysics and Biochemistry, Yale University, New Haven, Connecticut 06511, USA*

J. Lindenmann, *Institute for Immunology and Virology, University of Zürich, POB, CH-8028 Zürich, Switzerland*

T. C. Merigan, *Division of Infectious Diseases, Department of Medicine, Stanford University School of Medicine, Stanford, California 94305, USA*

F. H. Ruddle, *Department of Biology, Yale University, New Haven, Connecticut 06520, USA*

E. Saksela, *Department of Pathology, University of Helsinki, Finland*

D. L. Slate, *Department of Biology, Yale University, New Haven, Connecticut 06520, USA*

Y. H. Tan, *Department of Medical Biochemistry, University of Calgary, Calgary, Alberta T2N 1N4, Canada*

C. Weissmann, *Institut für Molekularbiologie I, Universität Zürich, 8093 Zürich, Switzerland*

Contents

Interferon and Natural Killer Cells

Eero Saksela

Genetic Control of the Interferon System

Doris L. Slate, Frank H. Ruddle and Y. H. Tan

Mechanisms of Interferon Action: The $(2'-5')(A)_n$ Synthetase–RNase L Pathway

Peter Lengyel

The Cloning of Interferon and Other Mistakes

Charles Weissmann

Present Appraisal of and Future Hopes for the Clinical Utilization of Human Interferons

Thomas C. Merigan

The Role of Interferon in Natural Resistance

JEAN LINDENMANN

Institute for Immunology and Virology, University of Zürich, Zürich, Switzerland

I IN SEARCH OF HEALTH

Medicine purports to maintain or restore health. An uncommitted observer from some distant planet might therefore expect biomedical research to be mainly directed at investigating health. Strangely enough this is not so: biomedical research is primarily concerned with disease.

It is true that physiology aims at elucidating normal function but it does so under highly abnormal conditions. Health is not simply an accretion of normal functions but the continuing effort to stabilize a permanently threatened equilibrium. Of course examples of such dynamic equilibria abound and physiology itself presents us with many. Thus, the seemingly static posture of a man standing upright can be dissected into its elements of motion and countermotion. In this case analysis is easy because the main force which impinges on the equilibrium, gravity, is known and constant.

When we come to the dynamic equilibrium we call health, we are quite ignorant of the actual stresses with which it has to cope. Some can be guessed, such as loss or accumulation of heat. Others may be surmised, like the ageing and functional degradation of certain cells or molecules. Still other possible disturbances are entirely hypothetical: do we have to imagine our skin and mucous membranes as the site of a never-ending struggle between defence mechanisms and malevolant intruders, our inner organs as battle-grounds where malignant cells are ever so often summarily despatched?

With respect to any given disturbance, an equilibrium has a certain range within which regulation occurs and beyond which it breaks down. When disease is being studied, interest is focused on events past the breakdown point. In the field of experimental infection, conditions are usually so arranged that the result of intervention is reduced to a body count. Opposing forces at play before the breaking point is reached remain hidden. To reveal these forces, disturbances that stay well within the regulatory range have to be applied. However, in a well-tuned system like health the motions that re-establish balance are so swift and of such small amplitude that they can hardly be measured: rocking the equilibrium within its homoeostatic range does not result in any measurable reaction and it is therefore impossible to say whether the system is being rocked at all.

To give a simple example, if we apply a suspension of typhoid bacteria to healthy skin nothing happens. We may interpret this as showing that a tremendous challenge to our health, the encounter with fully virulent disease germs, has been successfully overcome by timely mobilization of protective forces. But we do not know if painting the skin with typhoid is in fact a challenge. To illustrate this point further: a car with pulled handbrake will not move when given either a longitudinal or a transverse push of a certain strength. But only the longitudinal push tests the quality of the breaks. In ignorance of the inner mechanics of the car, we would probably draw wrong conclusions from the observation that pushes in different directions yield the same result. Suppose now that certain types of cars were not fitted with handbrakes. These would show differences in stability depending on the direction of the push. From this we would learn that a longitudinal push truly challenges whatever opposes lengthwise movement in a parked car, whereas a transverse push would test a different mechanism.

Knowing now how to test longitudinal stability, we might try to damage certain systems in order to evaluate their role. The example I have chosen already gives an idea of the complexity to be expected: in the car fitted with a properly pulled handbrake, damaging clutch, gearbox, pistons or valves would hardly affect stability, but each of these manoeuvres would further destabilize the car without a handbrake. To see the function of the handbrake in a realistic perspective, as of major importance in preventing a parked car from rolling downhill but otherwise dispensable, would require a good deal of probing.

II GENETIC VARIANTS IN HOMOEOSTASIS

If we want to translate these simplistic considerations to the study of defence mechanisms operating in infectious diseases, we need the equivalent of cars of similar make, but with or without handbrakes, to know which challenges to apply. Most experimental infections have been selected to produce severe disease in laboratory animals; with respect to these infections laboratory animals behave like cars without handbrakes, and we have to look for the occasional animal that withstands a usually lethal infection. The reverse approach should also be successful, and there are examples from human pathology where the majority of people resist an infection and exceptional genotypes succumb to it. It is really an artefact of the experimental situation that leads to the impression that genetically determined susceptibility to an infectious disease is the rule and resistance is rare.

In the field of virology, the classical example of genetically determined resistance is that first observed 50 years ago by Sawyer and Lloyd (1931) and later extensively studied by the groups of Webster, Sabin and Koprowski (Bang, 1979). In this system various flaviviruses (formerly called arbor B viruses) will, when introduced by some appropriate route, kill the vast majority of inbred mice, but will spare members of some strains. That an adequate challenge is being applied is shown by the lethal effect on susceptible mice: the push is in the right direction to move the car. As to the mechanism which allows resistant mice to survive, isolating the equivalent of a handbrake has proved difficult, as can be surmised from the various explanations put forward by one and the same group over the years: thus, the immune system was implicated (Theis *et al.*, 1959); interferon was tentatively ruled out (Vainio *et al.*, 1961); cellular antibodies were suggested (Vainio and Koprowski, 1962); macrophages were thought important (Goodman and Koprowski, 1962); interferon temporarily gained favour (Hanson *et al.*, 1969); thermoregulation was implicated (Lagerspetz *et al.*, 1973) and dismissed (Darnell *et al.*, 1974); interferon was again pushed into the background with interfering viral particles now the primary suspects (Darnell and Koprowski, 1974; Brinton, 1981).

Hence a comparison between flavivirus-susceptible and flavivirus-resistant mice is not between cars with or without handbrakes, but more likely a comparison between a car with worn brake, clutch, gearbox and engine, and one where all these parts are in better shape.

III INBORN RESISTANCE TO ORTHOMYXOVIRUSES

A chance observation made in 1961 led to a model which may be unique in revealing the role of interferon. Mice of the inbred strain A2G proved resistant to intracerebral challenge with otherwise lethal amounts of neurotropic influenza A virus (Lindenmann, 1962). These mice have a strange history: they were thought to be descended from strain A, but fresh genetic material must have been introduced between 1942 and 1950 by an illegitimate mating. A2G indeed shares approximatively half of the alleles studied so far with A, and in particular the major histocompatibility configuration H-2^a (Lindenmann and Klein, 1967). Resistance is governed by a single, dominant gene: *Mx* (Lindenmann, 1964). Whereas homozygous *Mx/Mx* animals develop resistance within a few days of birth, heterozygous *Mx/*+ mice need longer to express resistance, depending somewhat on the challenge virus used. This shows how relative a term like "dominance" is: tested at, say, 5 days of age, resistance would appear to be recessive; at 5 weeks, dominant.

The difference between resistant and susceptible animals was not only seen upon intracerebral challenge with neurotropic virus, but also upon intranasal challenge with pneumotropic strains or intraperitoneal challenge with a hepatotropic strain. It was therefore felt that whatever caused resistance must be systemic and could not reside in some anatomical peculiarity of a single organ. The immune system, an obvious candidate, could be ruled out (Haller and Lindenmann, 1974; Fiske and Klein, 1975; Haller *et al.*, 1976). Macrophages expressed resistance *in vitro* when freshly prepared from the peritoneal cavity (Lindenmann *et al.*, 1978). However, upon prolonged cultivation all macrophages became uniformly susceptible. Macrophages taken from the peritoneal cavities of mice pretreated with anti-interferon serum were susceptible from the start (Haller *et al.*, 1979a). Whereas a causative role of macrophages in resistance became unlikely when bone marrow chimaeras between histocompatible resistant and susceptible mice proved to express the phenotype of the recipient and not that of the donor (Haller *et al.*, 1979b), the role of interferon had to be taken seriously. The arguments in favour of interferon as the crucial element in this form of resistance are the following:

1. Resistant animals treated with anti-interferon serum became fully susceptible (Haller *et al.*, 1979a).
2. Macrophages from resistant mice, which had become susceptible upon prolonged cultivation, could be rendered resistant to orthomyxoviruses by treatment with small doses of interferon. Macrophages from susceptible mice similarly treated remained unprotected (Haller *et al.*, 1980).
3. The same observation was also made with hepatocytes and embryonic fibroblasts from resistant and susceptible mice (Arnheiter *et al.*, 1980).
4. The differential effect of interferon on cells with or without *Mx* was only seen with orthomyxoviruses, but not with unrelated viruses such as EMC, VSV or herpes.

5. Newborn mice of genotype *Mx*/+, phenotypically susceptible during the first days of life, could be protected against lethal influenza virus challenge by small doses of interferon. Genotypically susceptible (+/+) newborn mice could not be similarly protected (Haller *et al.*, 1981a).
6. Disease produced in adult resistant animals by exceptional orthomyxovirus strains could be prevented by doses of interferon which were without effect on similarly infected susceptible mice (Haller *et al.*, 1981b).

This last point bears some elaboration. When the resistance spectrum of A2G mice was first established, we noted that resistance was manifested towards several influenza A and B strains and towards Sendai virus (Lindenmann *et al.*, 1963). Whether resistance against Sendai virus, a paramyxovirus, is dependent on the same gene has not been definitively settled; some degree of resistance to Sendai virus seems widespread (Stewart and Tucker, 1978). For the time being only resistance to strains of orthomyxoviruses can be firmly attributed to the gene *Mx*. However, even within the orthomyxo family some strains show a very large difference in pathogenic potential depending on presence or absence of *Mx*, whereas other strains show this to a lesser extent. A few strains, in fact, grow almost as well in *Mx*/*Mx* and +/+ mice and induce comparable pathology at the same virus dilutions. The first two strains seen to behave in this manner were both derived from A/Singapore/1/57 (Lindenmann *et al.*, 1963). These strains have been lost, and a later attempt at producing a mouse-adapted variant from a lyophilized ampoule of an early egg passage of the same strain yielded virus to which *Mx*-bearers were quite resistant. We therefore searched for other mouse-adapted strains labelled A/Singapore/1/57 and indeed found one which gave us the satisfaction of killing *Mx*/*Mx* mice as readily as +/+ mice. Detailed analysis of this strain revealed it as a close relative of A/PR/8/34, an old laboratory acquaintance. Other PR8 strains do show *Mx*-dependence, although sometimes not impressively. For instance, one PR8 virus tested originally reached almost the same endpoint titre on A2G and control mice, but at intermediary dilutions a prozone was observed in A2G mice only (Lindenmann *et al.*, 1963).

The availability of virus strains dependent or independent of *Mx* opens a new approach to the problem of resistance. Do these strains escape an interferon-induced antiviral state, or do they fail to induce interferon? The answer seems to be that they fail to induce interferon, for exogenously applied interferon does protect adult *Mx*/*Mx* mice; but a direct proof of defective interferon induction by these strains is still lacking. The prozone mentioned above could have been caused by a mixture of interferon-inducing and non-interferon-inducing virus.

IV THE COOPERATION BETWEEN *Mx* AND INTERFERON

How then does one account for resistance due to *Mx*? Cells possessing this allele are intrinsically as permissive for orthomyxoviruses as are cells devoid of it. Virus replication induces the formation of comparable amounts of interferon in both types of cells. This interferon in turn leads to antiviral states which are similar in both types of cells as far as viruses outside the orthomyxo group are concerned, but differ greatly when measured by challenge with influenza virus: in that case only cells equipped with *Mx* are extensively protected, whereas other cells remain susceptible. Macrophages from conventionally reared mice seem to enjoy a certain baseline level of "interferonization", which protects *Mx*-bearing macrophages even before their first encounter with virus. But this alone is not sufficient to protect the whole animal. Newborn mice are susceptible because they fail to produce sufficient amounts of interferon; given exogenous interferon, they are protectable according to their *Mx* status. Certain strains of virus apparently do not induce interferon and are therefore virulent for *Mx*-bearing mice; they can be held in check by exogenous interferon or interferon inducers.

Many interesting questions remain. How does spontaneous interferonization of macrophages come about and does it vary with age, diet, intestinal flora, subclinical infections, viral latency, carriage of endogenous viruses? How do certain virus strains avoid inducing interferon? And, perhaps the most interesting question: how does the *Mx* gene product collaborate with interferon to bring about an antiviral state which is spectacularly active against orthomyxoviruses?

On this last point I wish to indulge in some speculations. The *Mx* gene product is either constantly being made or it is switched on by interferon. If constantly present it could be an antiviral factor in its own right, blocking a metabolic pathway by which orthomyxovirus synthesis bypasses the interferon-induced antiviral state. Thus in cells lacking *Mx* interferon would be an inefficient inhibitor because orthomyxovirus synthesis would continue through the bypass channel, but in cells containing *Mx* the bypass channel would be permanently blocked, and interferon would be an efficient inhibitor. This is schematically illustrated in Fig. 1.

Another possibility would be for *Mx* to code for an interferon receptor. Suppose that different interferons induce different antiviral states which impinge more or less on different virus replication channels. IFN-x, for instance, would induce an antiviral state, blocking the orthomyxo replication channel, but to do so would require a receptor coded for by *Mx* (Fig. 2). This would require different receptors for different interferons, something which seems rather unlikely (Aguet and Blanchard, in press).

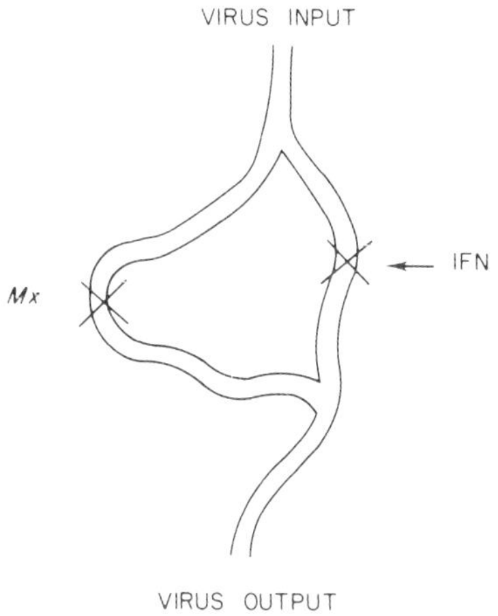

Fig. 1 Bypass hypothesis. In ordinary (+/+) mice interferon blockage of the usual replication channel for orthomyxoviruses (right channel) is bypassed (left channel). In *Mx*-bearing mice this bypass channel is permanently closed, and interferon is therefore a more efficient inhibitor of virus replication.

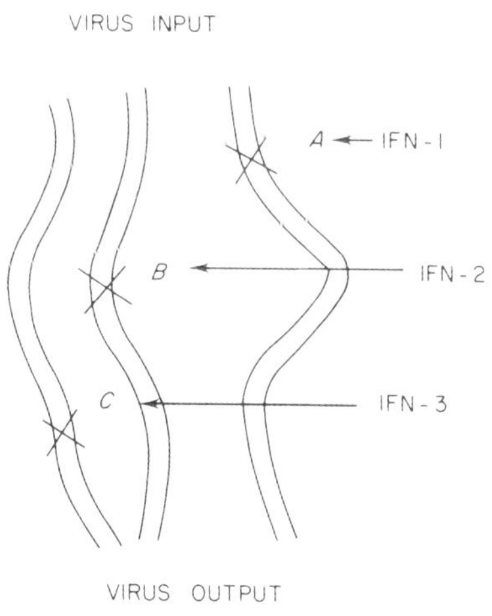

Fig. 2 Multiple interferon receptor hypothesis. The three paths represent independent replication channels for three groups of viruses. Genes *A, B, C* . . . each code for different receptors for interferons 1, 2, 3 . . . Each interferon induces an antiviral state which is specific for one replication channel only.

Lastly, the *Mx* gene product could be switched on only when interferon is present, and contribute to the antiviral state in such a manner as to render it efficient in blocking orthomyxoviruses (Fig. 3).

These three hypotheses, and several others that could be formulated, require that there be something unique in the replication of orthomyxoviruses—a channel distinct, at least at one point, from other replication channels through which other groups of viruses proceed. Advances in the clarification of the molecular biology of viruses should soon permit educated guesses as to what constitutes the sensitive event which is the target for the joint action of interferon and *Mx*.

That the ranking of viruses according to their interferon sensitivity depends on the test system used has long been recognized. Thus, vaccinia was the most interferon sensitive of five viruses in mouse and hamster cells, but the least interferon sensitive in rabbit cells (Stewart *et al.*, 1969). In these experiments both the cell type and the interferon preparation varied, which makes it difficult to decide which factor determined ranking. However, even within the same cell type, interferon sensitivity of different viruses varied with the degree of differentiation (Nilsen *et al.*, 1980). The antiviral state does not decay at the same speed for different viruses, and ranking may therefore depend on whether early yields or multiple viral cycles are being measured (Hallum *et al.*, 1970). Cell clones derived from the same origin have been described in which two viruses were similarly inhibited by interferon in one clone, and very dissimilarly in the other

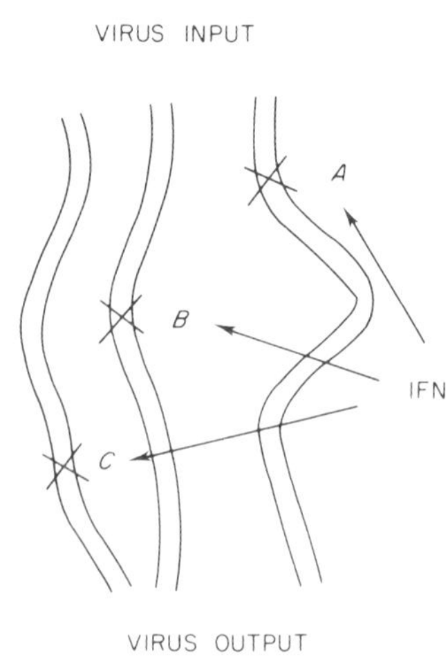

Fig. 3 Modulation of antiviral state hypothesis. The antiviral state is brought about by activation of genes *A, B, C* . . . each having its main effect on one replication channel only. Each channel allows replication of one group of viruses.

(Czarniecki *et al.*, 1981). Here the ranking is definitely dependent on the host cell.

In the *Mx* system very clear cut differences could be shown. Whereas in cells devoid of *Mx* influenza viruses can hardly be inhibited by interferon, in *Mx*-bearing cells they belong to the most interferon sensitive viruses. Depending on which cell is used very divergent opinions could be formed with respect to the interferon sensitivity of influenza virus. The same holds true for experiments *in vivo*: tested in *Mx*-bearing mice interferon would seem an efficient anti-influenza agent, and a very poor one in non-*Mx*-bearing mice. Such findings have obvious relevance for possible human applications of interferon.

V GENERAL IMPLICATIONS OF THE *Mx* SYSTEMS

Mx-governed resistance presents us with an example where interferon is the essential mediator. How far can such an insight be generalized? Obviously not by expecting that all instances of natural resistance will ultimately be reduced to the same mechanism. If interferon appears to be the dominating factor in resistance of mice to orthomyxoviruses, it is only an auxiliary factor in resistance to flaviviruses or in resistance to mouse hepatitis virus. That it plays a mitigating role within the more limited homoeostatic range of other virulent infections is seen from the effect of anti-interferon serum: infections with Semliki Forest, encephalomyocarditis, herpes simplex, Moloney sarcoma, vesicular stomatitis, Newcastle disease, polyoma, mouse hepatitis viruses all run a more severe course under anti-interferon globulin (Fauconnier, 1970; Gresser *et al.*, 1976a, b, 1979; Virelizier and Gresser, 1978). Interestingly, anti-interferon globulin was found not to alter influenza virus infection. Ordinary mice (i.e. lacking *Mx*) were employed in this study, suggesting that the mouse insensitive to interferon-mediated inhibition of influenza virus represents an exceptional state of affairs, and that the *Mx* carrier is more "natural".

That interferon cannot be held responsible for resistance in every case is most dramatically illustrated by those instances in which it contributes to pathogenesis: infection by lymphocytic choriomeningitis virus is rendered less severe by anti-interferon serum treatment (Rivière *et al.*, 1977; Gresser *et al.*, 1978). No sweeping statements are possible in this area, and each example deserves painstaking analysis. How complicated the situation really is becomes clear when the following facts are kept in mind: virus strains vary in their ability to induce interferon, and animals vary in their ability to respond to interferon-inducing stimuli (De Maeyer and De Maeyer-Guignard, 1979); virus strains also vary with respect to their interferon sensitivity, and this itself depends, as we have just seen, on the genetic make up of the host. Viral genome and host genome thus interact at two levels: interferon induction and interferon action. We do seem to have identified a handbrake, but many hands are fiddling around with it. The value of *Mx* as a model is not so much that it proves unequivocally that interferon can, within the proper genetic context, be a very efficient defence mechanism by itself; it suggests new approaches for the unravelling of those intracellular events which are triggered by interferon and which add up to what we still rather vaguely call the antiviral state. This will require quite an effort, though, and the time might be ripe for others to join in. It is strange that only one entirely independent group has attempted the study of *Mx* and appears to have soon abandoned it (Rusanova and Soloviev, 1966).

Inborn resistance of mice against influenza virus might easily have been discovered before 1950. Could this have led to an earlier discovery of interferon? Even with full knowledge of the interferon system its role in *Mx*-determined resistance was only realized after some 17 years, when potent anti-interferon serum had become available (Lindenmann, 1981). Of course it can be argued that knowledge of interferon, and particularly of its supposed lack of specificity, impeded rather than facilitated its acceptance as a factor in a form of resistance which was confined to one group of closely related viruses only. Perhaps a less prejudiced look would have shown the facts in their correct perspective much sooner. It is always difficult to figure things happening in a different order from the one we have come to accept as historical. Nevertheless, and although I have given some thought to this problem, I can hardly imagine reasonable experiments that could have been done and that would have led to interferon from an observation of *Mx*, although in principle this should have been possible. It is very disturbing to think that some facts we observe are linked with discoveries that lay in the future, but with connections of such subtlety that they defy our shrewdest guesses.

VI SUMMARY

Adult mice carrying the allele *Mx* are highly resistant against lethal infection by several strains of orthomyxoviruses. This resistance is mediated by interferon. In the presence of *Mx* interferon induces an antiviral state which is particularly effective in blocking orthomyxovirus replication. The relevance of these findings for maintenance of health are discussed.

VII ACKNOWLEDGEMENT

The work presented in this review was supported in part by the Swiss National Science Foundation (grants no. 3.139.077, 3.393.078 and 3.728.080).

VIII REFERENCES

Arnheiter, H., Haller, O. and Lindenmann, J. (1980). *Virology* **103**, 11–20.
Bang, F. B. (1978). *Adv. Virus Res.* **23**, 269–348.
Brinton, M. (1981). *In* "Natural Resistance to Tumors and Viruses" (Ed. O. Haller). Current Topics in Microbiology and Immunology, Vol. 92, pp. 1–14. Thieme, Stuttgart.
Czarniecki, C. W., Sreevalsan, T., Friedman, R. M. and Parret, A. (1981). *J. Virol.* **37**, 827–831.
Darnell, M. B. and Koprowski, H. (1974). *J. infect. Dis.* **129**, 248–256.
Darnell, M. B., Koprowski, H. and Lagerspetz, K. (1974). *J. infect. Dis.* **129**, 240–247.
De Maeyer, E. and De Maeyer-Guignard, J. (1979). *In* "Interferon 1979" (Ed. I. Gresser), pp 75–99. Academic Press, London and New York.
Fauconnier, B. (1970). *C. R. hebd. Acad. Sci., Paris* D **271**, 1464.
Fiske, R. A. and Klein, P. A. (1975). *Infect. Immun.* **11**, 576–587.
Goodman, G. T. and Koprowski, H. (1962). *Proc. Natn. Acad. Sci. U.S.A.* **48**, 160–165.
Gresser, I., Tovey, M. G., Bandu, M-T., Maury, C. and Brouty-Boyé, D. (1976a). *J. exp. Med.* **144**, 1305–1315.
Gresser, I., Tovey, M. G., Maury, C. and Bandu, M-T. (1976b). *J. exp. Med.* **144**, 1316–1323.
Gresser, I., Morel-Maroger, L., Verroust, P., Rivière, Y. and Guillon, J-C. (1978). *Proc. Natn. Acad. Sci. U.S.A.* **75**, 3413–3416.
Gresser, I., Maury, C., Kress, C., Blangy, D. and Maunoury, M-T. (1979). *Int. J. Cancer* **24**, 178–183.
Haller, O. and Lindenmann, J. (1974). *Nature, Lond.* **250**, 679–680.
Haller, O., Arnheiter, H. and Lindenmann, J. (1976). *Infect. Immun.* **13**, 844–854.
Haller, O., Arnheiter, H., Gresser, I. and Lindenmann, J. (1979a). *J. exp. Med.* **149**, 601–612.
Haller, O., Arnheiter, H. and Lindenmann, J. (1979b). *J. exp. Med.* **150**, 117–126.
Haller, O., Arnheiter, H., Lindenmann, J. and Gresser, I. (1980). *Nature, Lond.* **283**, 660–662.
Haller, O., Arnheiter, H., Gresser, I. and Lindenmann, J. (1981a). *J. exp. Med.* **154**, 199–203.
Haller, O., Arnheiter, H., Gresser, I. and Lindenmann, J. (1981b). *In* "The Biology of the Interferon System" (Eds E. de Maeyer, G. Galasso and H. Schellekens), pp. 187–191. Elsevier, Amsterdam.
Hallum, J. V., Thacore, H. and Youngner, J. S. (1970). *J. Virol.* **6**, 156–162.
Hanson, B., Koprowski, H., Baron, S. and Buckler, C. E. (1969). Microbios **1B**, 51–68.
Lagerspetz, K. Y. H., Koprowski, H., Darnell, M. and Tarkkonen, M. (1973). *Am. J. Physiol.* **225**, 532–537.
Lindenmann, J. (1981). *In* "Proceedings of the International Meeting on the Biology of the Interferon System" (Eds E. de Maeyer, G. Galasso and H. Schellekens), pp. 3–9. Elsevier, Amsterdam.
Lindenmann, J. (1962). *Virology* **16**, 203.
Lindenmann, J. (1964). *Proc. Soc. exp. Biol. Med.* **116**, 506–509.

Lindenmann J. and Klein, P. A. (1967). *In* "Recent Results in Cancer Research" (Ed. P. Rentchnick), Vol. 9. Springer-Verlag, Berlin, Heidelberg, New York.
Lindenmann, J., Lane, C. A. and Hobson, D. (1963). *J. Immunol.* **90**, 942–951.
Lindenmann, J., Deuel, E., Fanconi, S. and Haller, O. (1978). *J. exp. Med.* **147**, 531–540.
Nilsen, T. W., Wood, D. L. and Baglioni, C. (1980). *Nature, Lond.* **286**, 178–180.
Rivière, Y., Gresser, I., Guillon, J-C. and Tovey, M. G. (1977). *Proc. Natn. Acad. Sci. U.S.A.* **74**, 2135–2139.
Rusanova, N. A. and Soloviev, V. D. (1966). *Vopr. Virusol.* **11**, 398–402.
Sawyer, W. A. and Lloyd, W. (1931). *J. exp. Med.* **54**, 533–555.
Stewart, R. B. and Tucker, M. J. (1978). *Can. J. Microbiol.* **24**, 9–13.
Stewart, W. E., Scott, W. D. and Sulkin, S. E. (1969). *J. Virol.* **4**, 147–153.
Theis, G. A., Billingham, R. E., Silvers, W. K. and Koprowski, H. (1959). *Virology* **8**, 264–265.
Vainio, T. and Koprowski, H. (1962). *Acta path. microbiol. scand.* Suppl. **154**, 265.
Vainio, T., Gwatkin, R. and Koprowski, H. (1961). *Virology* **14**, 385–387.
Virelizier, J-L. and Gresser, I. (1978). *J. Immunol.* **120**, 1616–1619.

Interferon-Gamma: Is It Really Different from the Other Interferons?

LOIS B. EPSTEIN

Cancer Research Institute and Department of Pediatrics, University of California, San Francisco, California, USA

I INTRODUCTION

I first started working with IFN-γ while at the National Institutes of Health (NIH) in 1967. I had done some work several years previously with Fred Stohlman and George Brecher on the biochemical and morphological changes which occur when human lymphocytes are stimulated *in vitro* with phytohaemagglutinin (PHA) (Tanaka *et al.*, 1963; Epstein and Stohlman, 1964). When I joined Maurice Landy's Laboratory of Immunology I expanded these studies to include *in vivo* effects of PHA (Epstein and Smith, 1968). I was aware of Wheelock's report of an "interferon-like substance" in the supernatants of human leukocyte cultures stimulated with PHA (Wheelock, 1965), and so wrote to Tom Merigan whom I had met while he was at the NIH and asked whether he would be interested in examining the sera of PHA-treated mice for interferon. Thus started the collaborative effort which introduced me to the interferon field and allowed us, after I joined the faculty of the University of California at San Francisco, to continue with our studies of the cellular source of mitogen and antigen induced interferons (Epstein *et al.*, 1971a, b, 1972). I remember wondering why it took so long for other investigators to pick up on Wheelock's 1965 observation, which to me was fascinating. Friedman and Cooper did in 1967, and Green *et al.* in 1969, but for many years investigators in the field of interferon wondered why anyone, as I did, would bother with mitogens and antigens as inducers of interferon, especially since such low titres were observed and the interferon had much less stability to low pH and heat than did interferons induced by viruses. Similarly, cellular immunologists interested in products of lymphocytes and macrophages always wondered why I would bother working with interferon, as they would ask "what is the significance of the production of an antiviral substance during the course of an immune reaction to a nonviral antigen—what could it possibly mean?", and they would continue to list interferon at the bottom of the list of mediators of cellular immunity! I remember with what caution and restraint we suggested in a publication in 1971 that IFN-γ might have a regulatory role in the immune response:

> thus it is possible to envision that in the scheme of immunologic surveillance *in vivo* antigen induced interferon might have as many functions as have been ascribed to interferon induced by viral and other nonviral agents. Furthermore, the observation in the present study that the amount of antigen-induced interferon continues to increase as lymphocyte transformation declines suggests the intriguing possibility that interferon might be involved in the control of replication of normal cells, as well as parasites and tumor cells.
>
> (Epstein *et al.*, 1971b)

But now the tide has turned, perhaps too much, and there is tremendous interest, enthusiasm and expectation for the future of IFN-γ. Immunologists consider it of considerable potential as a biological response modifier, virologists and clinicians seek to exploit its potential as an antiviral agent, and oncologists yearn to use it as a new and possibly potent antitumour agent. In a recent programme on interferon televized both in the USA and elsewhere, a patient with malignancy who had received only little or no benefit from therapy with IFN-α was seen riding off in the distance in a taxi as the announcer extolled the hope and promise of IFN-γ in the future for the patient!

How did all this excitement arise? Part of it is due to the tremendous media campaign mounted by people interested in promulgating any kind of interferon as "the magic bullet" for the treatment of malignancy (*Time Magazine*, 1980). Interferon was portrayed as a natural product that had activity in only minute amounts and caused far less toxic and debilitating side effects than standard chemotherapeutic agents—but the publicity far outstripped the beneficial effects that were being observed. Furthermore there were a few reports that IFN-γ was more "potent" than the other interferons, and hence the heightened interest in that interferon class.

A few years ago I wrote a review entitled "The Comparative Biology of

Immune and Classical Interferons'' (Epstein, 1979) and the reader is referred to that review for progress up until that time. In that review I compared immune (or what is now known as IFN-γ) and classical interferons (or what are now known as IFN-α and IFN-β) with regard to various aspects of their production (i.e. inducers, cell source, mechanism of induction and genetic control), characterization, assay, mechanism of action, role as antiviral agents, effects on the immune response, other nonantiviral effects, clinical aspects of production, and use as therapeutic agents. Much more was known at that time (as is also the situation now) about classical interferon as it was described in 1957 (Isaacs and Lindenmann, 1957; Isaacs *et al.*, 1957) earlier than what was later called immune interferon, which was not described until 1965 (Wheelock, 1965). However, the information was sufficient to conclude that the immune system was the exclusive source of immune interferon but not of classical interferon, as a wide variety of cells in addition to the cells of the immune system, both *in vitro* and *in vivo*, have the capacity to produce classical interferon. Similarly, only a limited number of substances, i.e. mitogens, antigens, and allogeneic cells, were found to be capable of inducing immune interferon. By contrast, a wide variety of agents, including viruses and other intracellular microorganisms, products of bacteria, native and synthetic double stranded RNA, polymers and low molecular weight substances, are capable of inducing classical interferons.

We recognized then the heterogeneity of both classical and immune interferons as exemplified by their diversity of molecular weights, physical properties and antigenic configurations. We acknowledged that it was not at all clear how or whether the differences in physical properties between classical and immune interferons reflect differences in their molecular or antigenic configurations, range of antiviral activity, or spectrum of nonantiviral effects.

At that time studies to compare the biological effects of classical and immune interferon directly, and not with the aid of inducers, had been impeded by the lack of large quantities of high titred preparations of immune interferon. Investigators were forced, therefore, to use crude preparations, many of which contained numerous other lymphokines and factors that affected cell function independently of the action of interferon. Also, early attempts to partially purify immune interferon were complicated by the considerable loss of biological activity during the purification procedures. As a result, the production of antisera to immune interferon was somewhat delayed. Although it was well established that classical interferons had numerous effects on many components of the immune response as well as having many other diverse biologic effects, proof of such for immune interferon was slow in coming because of the lack of suitable preparations for study. It was quite clear early on, however, that both classical and immune interferons expressed their antiviral effects by conferring protection on cells against the challenge virus and not by a direct effect on the virus. And, it was clear that although originally defined as an antiviral substance, the antiviral function of all the interferons was only one among many properties of equal or greater importance. Finally, we raised the question as to whether immune and classical interferons represented different varieties of the same substance that have the same range of biologic effects, or whether they represented different substances with biologically distinct actions. On the basis of evidence available then we predicted that immune and classical interferons would prove to be variants of the same substance.

In view of the recent heightened interest in IFN-γ I was asked by the editors of this series to try to put all the recent information about IFN-γ into proper perspective. In attempting to do so I shall review our current state of knowledge on the similarities and differences between IFN-γ and the other interferons, give my thoughts as to the issue of relative potency and potential usefulness of each type and suggest rational reasons for continued basic and clinical research with IFN-γ.

II PURIFICATION AND STRUCTURE OF THE INTERFERONS

In the past four years there has been a virtual explosion in our knowledge concerning the structure of the interferons. The successful purification to homogeneity of human IFN-β (Knight, 1976; Tan *et al.*, 1979; Heine *et al.*, 1980), human IFN-α (Rubinstein *et al.*, 1979; Zoon *et al.*, 1979; Berg and Heron, 1980), and murine interferons (Knight, 1976; De Maeyer-Guignard *et al.*, 1978; Iwakura *et al.*, 1978; Kawakita *et al.*, 1978) was recognized as a signal achievement in view of the difficulties inherent in purifying proteins of such high specific activity and of limited source.

The amino acid composition of the human IFN-α and IFN-β were different (Rubinstein *et al.*, 1979; Tan *et al.*, 1979; Zoon *et al.*, 1979; Knight *et al.*, 1980), and differences were noted also between the two IFN-α preparations and the two IFN-β preparations.

Successful purification to homogeneity and amino acid composition studies were quickly followed by reports of partial amino acid sequences of the *N*-terminal portion of human IFN-β, of human lymphoblastoid (an IFN-α), three mouse interferons (Knight *et al.*, 1980; Taira *et al.*, 1980; Zoon *et al.*, 1980), and IFN-α from chronic myelogenous leukaemia cells (CML) (Levy *et al.*, 1980). As could be anticipated from the amino acid composition studies and from the observations that human IFN-α and IFN-β have different physical properties, host range, and dose response curves (Vilček *et al.*, 1977; Stewart, 1979), the *N*-terminal portions were nonidentical, as there was only one homologous amino acid in the first 13 amino acid residues. In contrast and somewhat unexpectedly, homology did exist at the *N*-terminal end of human lymphoblastoid and one of the mouse interferons (C) where 13 of 20 amino acids were identical. Also, three of 13 of IFN-β and another mouse interferon (A) were identical. The sequence reported for IFN-α derived from CML cells (Levy *et al.*, 1980) was identical to that observed with IFN-α from lymphoblastoid cells (Zoon *et al.*, 1980) for the first 20 amino acids with only two exceptions. Thus numerous authors agreed upon the heterogeneity of the primary structure of human IFN-α and the marked divergence of primary structure between IFN-α and IFN-β.

A giant leap forward for the field of interferon occurred when recombinant DNA technology was employed for the cloning of the gene for human IFN-β (Derynck *et al.*, 1980a, b; Taniguchi *et al.*, 1980a, b) and several genes for IFN-α (Goeddel *et al.*, 1980a, b, 1981; Maeda *et al.*, 1980; Nagata *et al.*, 1980a, b; Streuli *et al.*, 1980). Recombinant DNA technology potentially permits the production of various interferons in unlimited quantities and has provided profound insights into the comparative primary structure of the various interferons, their genetic control, evolutionary history and the influence of primary structure on function and physical properties. When one pools the data from the published and as yet unpublished recombinant DNA information presented at a recent meeting in Rotterdam on the biology of the interferon system (Weissmann, personal communication, 1981) with data arrived at by independent techniques [i.e. amino acid analysis of tryptic and chymotryptic peptides of lymphoblastoid interferon (IFN-α) (Allen and Fantes, 1980) and by techniques for the sequencing of cDNA for IFN-β (Houghton *et al.*, 1980)] the following becomes apparent. First, at least 12 genes have been found which code for human IFN-α and the nucleotide sequence of these is known. The nucleotide sequences demonstrate that the genes for IFN-α code for a family of homologous proteins, distinct from each other by less than 20% of their 165 or 166 amino acids. In contrast, the homology between human IFN-α and human IFN-β (also 166 amino acids long) is far less, as they are distinct from each other by more than 70% of their amino acids. The question as to whether there are multiple genes coding for human IFN-β, just as there are for IFN-α is yet to be resolved. Two, and more recently four populations of mRNA for human IFN-β have been described (Sehgal and Sagar, 1980; Sehgal, 1981).

Another major advance occurred with the development of monoclonal antibodies for human IFN-α (Secher and Burke, 1980; Staehelin *et al.*, 1981) and for human IFN-β (Hochkeppel *et al.*, 1981). Such is of immense importance for the rapid purification, development of radioimmunoassays (Secher, 1981), enzyme immunoassays, and for probing and confirming the structural nature and antigenic determinants of the various forms of the interferons.

Given the fact that human IFN-α exists in multiple forms governed by different genes (Nagata *et al.*, 1981), it is not unreasonable to conjecture that comparable multiple forms of IFN-γ exist. There is already information concerning the heterogeneity of IFN-γ (Osborne *et al.*, 1979, Wietzerbin *et al.*, 1979) but it is not known whether this results from the existence of multiple genes or from the post-translational modification of a single gene product. It is hoped that the many investigators who are working on the purification to homogeneity of IFN-γ, isolation of its mRNA, cloning of the gene or genes for IFN-γ will provide information in the future concerning this issue.

In the past few years considerable progress has been made in the purification of IFN-γ, as is depicted in Table I, but to date the specific activities have not reached that found for either pure IFN-α, [2·5 × 10^8 units/mg (Zoon *et al.*, 1979), 4·5 × 10^8 (Rubinstein *et al.*, 1979), or 10^9 (Berg and Heron, 1980)] or for pure human IFN-β [2 × 10^8 units/mg (Knight, 1976)]. Also, it is apparent from the data in Table I that the molecular weights found for IFN-γ are somewhat higher than the range observed for pure IFN-α (15 000–22 000) or IFN-β (20 000). It is possible that this might be due to a limited degree to glycosylation of the IFN-γ as it, like the other interferons, has been shown to be glycosylated (Mizrahi *et al.*, 1978). But, after mild SDS treatment of HuIFN-γ, molecular weight forms of 20 000 and 25 000 have recently been observed (Yip and Vilček, personal communication, 1981). Also, like the situation with the recombinant DNA forms of IFN-α (Marcucci *et al.*, 1980), and IFN-β (Derynck *et al.*, 1980a) and lymphoblastoid interferon (Allen and Fantes, 1980), or the mouse interferons (Fujisawa *et al.*, 1978; Havell and Carter, 1981) the glycosylation of IFN-γ is not necessary for either its production or its antiviral action (Mizrahi *et al.*, 1978). Similarly, both mouse IFN-γ and the other mouse interferons share a polynucleotide binding site (De Maeyer-Guignard *et al.*, 1977; Wietzerbin *et al.*, 1978a). In view of the fact that IFN-γ has been shown to have the same actions as the other interferons, as will be discussed below, I would predict that although it can exist as a larger molecule, that considerable homology with the other interferons will be found, especially in critical areas of the molecule involved in specific functions.

Antibodies to IFN-γ have helped to characterize further preparations of this interferon produced in response to different inducers. For example, Osborne *et al.* (1980) found that a rabbit antiserum to SEA induced murine IFN-γ, neutralized IFN-γ induced *in vitro* by SEA, Con A, PHA-P and PWM, and IFN produced as a result of mixed lymphocyte culture. In addition, it neutralized the IFN-γ produced *in vivo* by mice sensitized with BCG and challenged with OT. Similar results were observed

Species	Cell source	Inducer	Method of purification	pI	Specific activity (units/mg)	Mol. wt	Reference
Human	Peripheral blood mono-nuclear cells	SEA	Chromatography on controlled pore glass (CPG) and poly U agarose	8·3	5×10^{7}	—	Sedmak *et al.* personal communication, 1981)
Human	Peripheral blood mono-nuclear cells	SEA	PEG precipitation, chromatography on DEAE Sepharose; adsorption on SP—Sephadex, Ultragel Ac 44	—	10^{7}	50 000	Koistinen and Cantell (1981)
Human	Peripheral blood mono-nuclear cells	TPA and PHA	Chromatography on CPG and Con A Sepharose and Biogel 200	8·6	10^{7}	58 000 (± 3 000)	Yip *et al.* (1981)
Human	Peripheral blood lymphocytes	PHA or Con A	Chromatography on Con A Sepharose, gel filtration and anti BSA Sepharose	4·0–4·5	10^{6}	36 000	Sato and Yamane (1981)
Human	Peripheral blood mono-nuclear cells	PHA	Chromatography on CPG and poly U agarose	—	10^{6}	—	Wiranowska-Stewart *et al.* (1980)
Human	Peripheral blood mono-nuclear cells	Con A	Batch adsorption on CPG	—	$10^{5 \cdot 3}$	45 000	de Ley *et al.* (1980)
Human	Peripheral blood mono-nuclear cells	SEA	Adsorbed with Matrex Blue; chromatography on CPG Ultragel AcA 54	4·0–4·3; 4·91–5·38	$10^{6 \cdot 3}$	35–70 000	Georgiades *et al.* (1979); Goldstein *et al.* (1979)
Mouse	Spleen cells	SEA	NH_4SO_4; chromatography on BSA-Affigel or hydroxyl-apatite, Ultragel AcA 34	—	—	40 000 70 000–90 000	Osborne *et al.* (1980)
Mouse	Spleen cells	PHA	Chromatography on Con A Sepharose, Affigel 202, Blue Sepharose CL 6B, phenyl Sepharose CL 4B	—	—		Wietzerbin *et al.* (1979)

by Stefanos *et al.*, (1980) who found that rabbit antiserum to PHA induced murine IFN-γ neutralized IFN-γ produced *in vitro* in response to PHA, Con A and Suc Con A. Their data indicated that preparations of IFN-γ produced under diverse conditions are antigenically the same or closely related. The same situation pertains to human IFN-γ, as preparations induced by SEA, PHA-M, Con A and PWM, galactose oxidase and calcium ionophore were neutralized by a rabbit antiserum to SEA induced human IFN-γ (Langford *et al.*, 1981). Of interest was the observation that all of these antisera to IFN-γ did not neutralize either virus induced IFN-α or IFN-β. In fact, one was useful in confirming that preparations of PHA-P induced IFN-γ are contaminated by other interferons and that IFN-α appears to contaminate the IFN-γ produced by sensitized lymphocytes in response to PPD (Langford *et al.*, 1981). Other investigators have also reported that preparations of SEA, PHA or PWM induced human IFN-γ are contaminated with IFN-α (Wiranowska-Stewart, 1981), *Corynebacterium parvum* induced IFN-γ is contaminated with IFN-α (Vilček *et al.*, 1980) or a form of IFN intermediate between γ and α (Epstein *et al.*, 1980b), and preparations of Con A induced IFN-γ are contaminated with IFN-β (de Ley *et al.*, 1980). There is already precedent in the literature for the production of two types of interferons in response to a single inducer, in that both IFN-α and IFN-β are produced by human fibroblasts in response to NDV (Hayes *et al.*, 1979) and this has been confirmed by isolating mRNA for both interferons from the fibroblasts (Pang *et al.*, 1980).

Several laboratories have already isolated and translated the mRNA for HuIFN-γ (Taniguchi *et al.*, 1981; Wallace *et al.*, 1981; Billiau *et al.*, personal communication, 1981). These studies thus pave the way for future production of IFN-γ by recombinant DNA techniques.

III INDUCERS AND CELL SOURCE

A wide variety of substances induce IFN-α and IFN-β, and these have been classified recently as to their potency (Baron *et al.*, 1979). However we still do not know what common or dissimilar mechanisms exist whereby they all are able to induce interferon. Far fewer substances are known to induce IFN-γ, including mitogens, bacterial and viral antigens, allogeneic cells, and antisera directed against surface components. For example, murine OKT3 monoclonal antibody which reacts with human mature T cells induces the production of IFN-γ in cultured mononuclear cells (Chang *et al.*, 1981; Wussow *et al.*, 1981), whereas OKT4 which reacts with the helper population and OKT8 which reacts with the suppressor T cell subset do not. Although the inducers of IFN-γ are diverse in nature and composition, a common feature is that they all appear to interact with various components of the cell surface. The development of antisera to the various interferons has permitted characterization of the interferons produced in response to a given agent. Such studies have confirmed that a given inducer can stimulate the production of more than one type of interferon, as NDV has been shown to induce both IFN-α and IFN-β from human fibroblasts (Pang *et al.*, 1980), PHA induces IFN-γ and IFN-α from peripheral blood mononuclear cells (Wiranowska-Stewart, 1981) and Con A induces IFN-γ and IFN-β from the same cells (de Ley *et al.*, 1980). Furthermore, agents which were thought previously to be exclusively inducers of IFN-γ, such as PPD, are now known to induce other interferons as well (Langford *et al.*, 1981).

We hoped we were making an important contribution to the field of interferon research when we found that lymphocytes could produce IFN-γ in response to mitogens and specific bacterial and viral antigens (Epstein *et al.*, 1971a, b, 1972). In the early days of doing cell source studies antisera to the various interferons were not available for precise characterization of the interferons produced in response to a given agent and we had to rely on the lability to heating at 56°C and treatment at pH 2 to identify IFN-γ.

Soon it was realized that lymphocytes could be separated into two classes: T or thymic derived cells or B or bone marrow derived cells. We wished to ascertain which would be the source of IFN-γ and found in fact that both cell types produced IFN and required the presence of macrophages for maximum interferon production (Epstein *et al.*, 1974). Soon afterwards it was found that T lymphocytes could be further separated into subclasses depending on the receptors on their surfaces for the Fc portion of immunoglobulins. We thus proceeded to study the production of IFN-γ by T_μ, T_γ, and T_ϕ cells and found that all three subclasses produced it in response to PHA and that macrophages enhanced the production of each subset (Epstein and Gupta, 1981). In the mouse Archer *et al.* (1979) had also found that more than one type of T cell subpopulation was capable of producing IFN-γ. SEA induced it primarily in T_1 cells (cells of recent thymic origin, shortlived and nonrecirculating), PHA primarily in T_2 cells (cells containing both suppressor, helper and memory functions) and Con A in both T_1 and T_2 cells.

And would you believe it? There are now thought to be subclasses of the subclasses of human and mouse T lymphocytes as defined by specific antigens on their surface but we will encourage others to take over where we left off with regard to cell source studies! For example, Landolfo *et al.* (1981) just defined the phenotype of T cells which produce IFN-γ in the primary mixed lymphocyte culture as a Lyt 1^+, Qat 5^+ and Lyt 123^+, Qat 5^+, and those in the secondary mixed lymphocyte culture as Lyt 1^+, Qat 5^+; Lyt 123^+, Qat 5^+; and Lyt 23^+, Qat 5^-. One could potentially spend a lifetime refining the cellular source of interferon as new reagents to define cell surface antigens become available! I do not mean to make light of our own previous studies on cell source or those of others, as they are of critical importance in understanding the surface molecules on lymphocytes and lymphocyte–interferon inducer interactions.

Obviously, the critical point in all of the studies which have been performed by many investigators is the purity of the cell suspensions employed. One cannot, for example, make definitive statements in good conscience about monocytes as a cell source of IFN-γ, as has been done recently, when they contain 20% of nonmonocyte cells as assessed by a nonspecific esterase stain. It has been suggested that only 0·1% of the total mononuclear population makes α interferon and only 0·1% of T cells make IFN-γ in response to PHA (Wiranowska-Stewart and Stewart, 1981). If this is substantiated in the future by the work of other laboratories, then the question of the adequacy of cell separation techniques and resultant purity of subpopulations under study assumes even greater importance than thought previously.

As the subject of cell source of IFN-γ has recently been reviewed (Epstein, 1978, 1982), I would refer the reader to those reviews for a summary of cell sources found for each inducer studied. What would seem most appropriate for the remainder of this section would be to review the important conclusions and recent advances concerning cell source of IFN-γ, particularly as they relate to either similarities or differences from the other interferons.

The range of cell types producing IFN-γ is more narrow than that which produces the other interferons. IFN-γ is produced by cells of the immune system (T and B lymphocytes) and the interaction of such cells with macrophages is required for the production in response to certain inducers (i.e. PHA, PWM, PPD) but not to others [*C. parvum* (Sugiyama and Epstein, 1978), and a protein from *Staphylococcus aureus* (Ratcliff *et al.*, 1981)]. However, lymphocytes and cells of the monocyte–macrophage lineage are also capable of producing IFN-α (for review, see Lucas and Epstein, 1981). Human B lymphocytes produce IFN-α in response to xenogeneic or allogeneic tumour cells (Weigent *et al.*, 1981), and null lymphocytes produce it in response to tumour cells, HSV and *C. parvum* (Peter *et al.*, 1980). Using fluorescence microscopy with the first monoclonal antibody to human IFN-α, Secher and Cantell (personal communication, 1981) have found that monocytes are the source of Sendai virus induced IFN-α, the same IFN-α which has been used in therapeutic trials for malignancy and infectious diseases in man. Human macrophages produce IFN-α in response to influenza virus (Roberts *et al.*, 1979) and to herpes simplex virus infected cells (Stanwick *et al.*, 1981). Spontaneous production by Ia negative macrophages has also been noted (Ito *et al.*, 1981). Thus to date, cells which produce IFN-γ have the capacity to produce other interferons, but cells like fibroblasts and epithelial cells which produce both IFN-β and IFN-α have been found not to produce IFN-γ. A monoclonal antibody to HuIFN-γ has recently been reported (Hochkeppel *et al.*, personal communication, 1981). Once it becomes readily available, the nature and proportion of cells which produce IFN-γ in response to a given inducer in normal and disease states can be elucidated more precisely.

With a multiplicity of investigators working in the field, former beliefs are now being challenged. For example, it was previously believed that only sensitized lymphocytes responded to specific antigens with the production of IFN-γ. Recently, Lee *et al.* (1981) found that high doses of PPD induced IFN-γ and IFN-α in both sensitized and nonsensitized B lymphocytes. Nonsensitized and sensitized lymphocytes have also been shown to respond to specific antigens, i.e. PPD (Langford *et al.*, 1981) and a crude CMV antigen preparation (Starr *et al.*, 1980) with the production of IFN-α. However, in the latter situation when a purified CMV antigen was employed only cultures obtained from seropositive donors produced interferon, and it was predominantly of the IFN-γ type (Starr *et al.*, 1980).

Nevertheless there are numerous recent reports which substantiate the early observations that IFN-γ production is primarily a T lymphocyte dependent function (Kirchner *et al.*, 1979). IFN-γ can be produced by murine T cell clones derived from longterm culture, and IFN-γ is produced after the interaction of T lymphocytes and allogeneic cells (Ito *et al.*, 1979, 1980; Perussia *et al.*, 1980) and T lymphocytes and mycoplasma infected tumour cells (Beck *et al.*, 1980). Studies in nude mice in which IFN-γ was induced by PHA (Wietzerbin *et al.*, 1978b) but not by Con A (Kirchner *et al.*, 1980) or allogeneic cells (Kirchner *et al.*, 1979) suggest that a different cell source might obtain for each inducer.

Whereas T cell–allogeneic cell interactions result in IFN-γ production, T cell–tumour cell interactions result in IFN-α production. The preponderance of evidence suggests that cells which spontaneously kill allo- or xenogeneic targets, called natural killer (NK) cells, are in the T cell lineage (Herberman, 1980) and that growth factors produced in culture promote their differentiation (Kraft *et al.*, 1981; Ortaldo *et al.*, 1981). The production of IFN-α by NK cells in contact with their tumour targets has been demonstrated by several groups (Timonen *et al.*, 1980; Trinchieri *et al.*, 1980; Djeu *et al.*, 1981). Further exploration of this system should provide considerable practical information concerning lymphocyte–tumour cell interactions; it represents another example of how cells in the T cell lineage, which have the capacity to produce IFN-γ, also produce IFN-α.

It has been suggested that the production of IFN-γ requires T lymphocytes, alloantigen, and interleukin II (formerly known as T cell growth factor) (Farrar *et al.*, 1981). The interdependence of IFN-γ, the cells which produce it, and other mediators of cellular immunity or biological response modifiers, such as thymic extracts (Shoham *et al.*, 1980), should provide fertile ground for future investigators.

Defects in IFN-γ production have already been found in certain patients with selective IgA deficiency (Epstein and Ammann, 1974), chronic lymphocytic leukaemia (Epstein and Cline, 1974), two patients with partial albinism with impairment of phagocytosis, one with a lupus-like syndrome, and one patient with multiple infections with splenomegaly (Lipinski *et al.*, 1980), persistent Epstein-Barr virus infection with hypergammaglobulinaemia (Virelizier *et al.*, 1978) and in normal cord blood samples (Bryson *et al.*, 1980). Hopefully it will be possible in the future to determine when depressed IFN-γ production reflects an absent or functionally defective cell population, or absence of factors, such as interleukin II, which have been suggested to influence its production.

IV ACTIONS OF INTERFERONS

How lucky it was for those of us in the field of interferon research that so many of the biologic effects of interferon that were determined by the use of crude or partially purified preparations were confirmed once interferon was purified to homogeneity! Electrophoretically pure mouse interferon was shown to inhibit the growth of a transplantable tumour (Erlich ascites tumour) *in vivo*, to inhibit the multiplication of L 1210 tumour cells *in vitro*, to enhance the expression of histocompatibility antigens on mouse L 1210 cells *in vitro*, to inhibit antibody formation *in vitro*, to inhibit the sensitization to sheep erythrocytes and the expression of delayed type hypersensitivity in mice, to enhance NK activity *in vivo* and *in vitro*, to enhance the sensitivity of cells to the toxicity of poly I: poly C, and to enhance production of interferon by priming (Gresser *et al.*, 1979). The biologic properties of the pure interferons have recently been reviewed by Knight (1980), and extensive reviews on the effects of interferons on cell growth and functions (Taylor-Papadimitriou, 1980) and on the immune response *in vivo* and *in vitro* (Epstein, 1977; Sonnenfeld, 1980) also exist.

Since these articles were written it also has become clear that the interferons produced by recombinant DNA technology are biologically active *in vivo* and *in vitro*. Cloned preparations of IFN-α have antiviral activity *in vivo* (Goeddel *et al.*, 1980b) and *in vitro* (Nagata *et al.*, 1980), and so does cloned IFN-β (Derynck *et al.*, 1980b; Taniguichi *et al.*, 1980a). Also, the first IFN-α cloned by Charles Weissmann and his colleagues (α_1) has been shown to share with natural IFN-α the ability to enhance NK activity of lymphocytes, to enhance antibody dependent cell-mediated cytotoxicity, to suppress antigen and mitogen induced inhibition of leukocyte migration and to inhibit the growth of Burkitt lymphoma cells (Masucci *et al.*, 1980).

Also, it is now clear that the multiple forms of IFN-α produced by recombinant DNA technology have distinct functional properties (Streuli *et al.*, 1980), and major differences in the antiviral activities on cells of different species (Goeddel *et al.*, 1981). It is most likely that these functional differences reflect differences in the primary, secondary or tertiary structure of the interferons and how each interferon interacts with the cell membrane and cytoskeleton of the cells in the various test systems (Pfeffer *et al.*, 1980; Bourgeade *et al.*, 1981; Chany, 1981).

If we turn to the literature on the biology of IFN-γ it is not surprising that it has been difficult to relate the work from one laboratory to that of another. Studies published to date have employed either crude or partially purified preparations of IFN-γ and some of these have been shown to contain contaminants of IFN-α (Wiranowska-Stewart, 1981) or IFN-β (de Ley *et al.*, 1980). Invariably, experimental protocols differ with regard to either the inducing agents, origin or composition of the leukocyte populations induced, purity of the resulting IFN-γ preparations, target cells for antiviral and functional assays, challenge viruses and method of quantitation of the assays. Also investigators are working very hard to produce a well standardized, stable international standard for IFN-γ with which the results of assays performed in different laboratories can be compared, but at the present time this is not yet available (Grossberg, personal communication, 1981). Hopefully it soon will be possible to analyse the properties of IFN-γ as a pure defined substance or family of pure substances. In the meantime using the data that are available in the literature we can give our thoughts on what appears to be a crucial question for IFN-γ: "does it have any unique biologic effects as compared with IFN-α or IFN-β?" At the present time there is no evidence that IFN-γ has any unique effects on normal cell functions. The range of actions of IFN-γ appears to be the same as for the other interferons and includes antiviral effects as well as the ability to enhance NK activity (de Ley *et al.*, 1980; Senik *et al.*, 1980), depress the antibody response to SRBC (Sonnenfeld *et al.*, 1977), inhibit the proliferation of nonmalignant (Blalock *et al.*, 1980; Rubin and Gupta, 1980) and malignant cell lines (de Ley *et al.*, 1980; Hovanessian *et al.*, 1980a; Rubin and Gupta, 1980), and tumours (Crane *et al.*, 1978), induce specific peptides (Hovanessian *et al.*, 1980b; Rubin and Gupta, 1980; L. B. Epstein *et al.*, 1981) and enzymes [$(2'p5'A)_n$ synthetase and protein kinase] (Hovanessian *et al.*, 1980a, b) and transfer resistance to viruses across species (Blalock *et al.*, 1979). There are special circumstances in experiments which employ L 1210 cells resistant to IFN-α and IFN-β in which IFN-γ is still active and IFN-α and IFN-β are not (Hovanessian *et al.*, 1980a), but these situations might be explained in terms of a mutation in the responding cells, rather than a unique function for IFN-γ. Obviously, as was the case with IFN-α and IFN-β, studies to confirm the range of actions of IFN-γ must be repeated once the pure material becomes available.

V POTENCY OF INTERFERONS

To my knowledge, the first allusion to the high potency of IFN-γ was made by Salvin *et al.* (1975). In their studies they used serum from tuberculin sensitive mice which had been challenged with old tuberculin (OT) as a source of IFN-γ. Daily injections of 300 units of this material for 3–4 weeks into mice bearing a transplantable, 3-methylcholanthrene-induced sarcoma (MC 36) resulted in 98% inhibition of tumour growth. The investigators recognized that their IFN-γ preparations also contained numerous other lymphokines which could have interacted synergistically with the IFN-γ or have affected the tumours either directly or indirectly via their effects on the immune system. Nevertheless, they still alluded to the potency of IFN-γ pointing out that in studies of other investigators (Gresser and Bourali, 1970) that far more virus induced interferon (i.e. 20 000 units/d for 1–2 months) was necessary to increase the survival time of mice challenged with other types of tumours (i.e. Erlich ascites, RC 19, and L 1210 leukaemia).

Using similar serum preparations which contained IFN-γ as well as numerous other lymphokines, and also a partially purified IFN-γ preparation, Sonnenfeld *et al.* (1977) found that the IFN-γ preparations were 250 times more active than a virus induced interferon in suppressing the murine antibody response to SRBC *in vivo* and *in vitro.* The antiviral potency of the interferon preparations, and hence their unitage was established on L 929 cells by a virus plaque reduction technique with VSV. The *in vivo* studies on antibody production were performed with Swiss Webster mice and the *in vitro* studies with BALB/c spleen cells.

Crane *et al.* (1978) also used lymphokine containing OT stimulated mouse serum as a source of IFN-γ and compared this with a crude NDV induced murine interferon for their antitumour effect against a transplantable murine osteogenic sarcoma line in C57BL/6 mice. Basing the amount of the two interferons employed on their antiviral activity against VSV challenged L 929 cells, the investigators found that inhibition of tumour development was achieved with 100 times less IFN-γ than that required for the virus induced interferon.

In other studies, an osteogenic sarcoma line, HeLa cells and a transformed U amnion cell line were found *in vitro* to be more sensitive to the growth inhibitory properties of a partially purified preparation of SEA induced human IFN-γ (specific activity $10^{4.5}$units/mg) than they were to pure human fibroblast interferon (Rubin and Gupta, 1980). The amounts of the two interferons employed were determined by their antiviral titre on human fibroblasts challenged with VSV.

These investigators noted greater sensitivity of reovirus and vaccinia to IFN-γ than was observed to IFN-β, whereas the replication of VSV and

EMC viruses were inhibited more strongly by IFN-β. In yet another system, a SEA induced murine IFN-γ was reported to be 3–10 times more efficient than crude virus induced L cell interferon in transferring resistance to viruses across species. The amounts of the interferons employed were determined by their antiviral effects against VSV (Blalock *et al.*, 1979).

Thus, as can be seen from the aforementioned studies, IFN-γ has been reported to be more potent than the other interferons for its immunoregulatory, antitumour and antiviral actions. In contrast, however, are several other studies which indicate that the immunoregulatory (de Ley *et al.*, 1980; Falcoff *et al.*, 1980), antitumour (de Ley *et al.*, 1980) and antiviral (Bourgeade *et al.*, 1980) effects are less or equipotent to those of IFN-α and IFN-β.

There is some important additional information in the literature which is helpful in resolving the question of relative potencies of the various interferons. First of all, some IFN-γ preparations have been shown to be contaminated with IFN-α (Wiranowska-Stewart, 1981) or IFN-β (de Ley *et al.*, 1980), and IFN-γ and IFN-β have been shown to potentiate the antiviral (Fleischmann *et al.*, 1979) and antitumour effects (Fleischmann *et al.*, 1980) of each other. Thus, unless the preparations used for comparison are well characterized with regard to extent of contamination with other interferons or other lymphokines, the estimates of IFN-γ content might be imprecise. Furthermore, all of the studies on comparative potency use amounts of IFN-α or β and IFN-γ that give equivalent antiviral effects, with the assumption that cells used in the antiviral assay recognize IFN-γ as well as they recognize the other interferons. We now know that this is not true, and that in fact, different cells respond in varying degrees to the various interferons. It has been the experience of several laboratories, depending on how and with what target cells the IFN-γ is assayed, that the relative potencies of IFN-α, IFN-β, and IFN-γ are different.

In Table II are depicted the preliminary results of a collaborative effort between my own laboratory and that of Dr Sidney Grossberg which illustrates this point. It is clear that our diploid fibroblasts do not recognize the antiviral potency of human IFN-γ as well as they recognize that of human IFN-β or α. Furthermore, the aneuploid A 549 lung cancer line apparently recognizes all the interferons equally well. Thus if we were to use our antiviral assay on diploid fetal lung fibroblasts to find comparable doses of IFN-γ and IFN-α, far more IFN-γ would be used. If these interferon preparations were then tested for antitumour potency on A 549 cells in these apparently "equal" amounts, the IFN-γ would appear to be a much more potent antitumour agent than IFN-α. Thus, it would be more accurate to test antiviral efficacy on the same cells as to be tested for antitumour or immunoregulatory properties, but this can not always be and was not achieved in most of the studies in which relative potency was under study.

TABLE II Comparison of Antiviral Activities of Human Interferons on Different Human Cell Strains

	Interferon Titre[a]		
	Diploid fetal lung fibroblasts	Trisomic fetal lung fibroblasts	Aneuploid carcinoma of lung
NIH Standard IFN-α	24 000	360 000	20 000
NIH Standard IFN-β	1 400	4 900	10 000
SEA induced IFN-γ internal laboratory standard	1 400	6 200	30 000

[a] Interferon assayed by EMC-HA yield reduction assay with 70% inhibition as the endpoint (Jameson and Grossberg, 1979) at the Medical College of Wisconsin.

Furthermore, as we lack an international interferon standard for IFN-γ, one man's unit might be another man's megaunit depending on the cells used in the assay, and the endpoint of the assay. At the present time all units for IFN are arbitrary and will be until such time when pure IFN is obtained, and activity is converted to molar amounts. Once pure IFN-γ preparations produced in response to a variety of inducers are obtained, they can be accurately and precisely compared as to potency, microgram for microgram, with regard to each other and with regard to IFN-α and IFN-β, for all their known biologic effects. Hopefully, the issue of comparative potency will be definitively resolved in the near future.

VI GENETIC CONTROL AND RESPONSE MECHANISMS

Although the gene for the production of human IFN-β was originally assigned to human chromosomes 2 and 5 (Tan *et al.*, 1974; Morgan and Faik, 1977; Tan, 1977; Slate and Ruddle, 1979a), more recent evidence indicates that chromosome 9 is also (Slate and Ruddle, 1980) or exclusively involved (Meager *et al.*, 1979; Burke, 1980; Burke and Meager, 1980). Confirmation of the latter was provided by Owerback *et al.* (1981) who localized to chromosome 9 not only the human IFN-β gene but also at least eight human IFN-α genes. In addition, some of the genes for IFN-α are closely linked as Nagata *et al.* (1980a) have identified two α clones which contained two linked genes each, and Lawn *et al.* (1981) have found one α clone which contains two IFN-α genes which lack intervening sequences and are separated by 12 kilobases, and Ullrich *et al.* (1981) have found another with two other IFN-α genes that are only five kilobases apart.

In the mouse another set of genetic loci have been described which influence the production of interferon, but how these relate to the situation known in man is not known (De Maeyer and De Maeyer-Guignard, 1979). The loci, called If-1, If-2, If-3 and If-4, are virus specific for induction of interferon by NDV, murine MTV, and Sendai virus, respectively. They control the ability of various mouse strains to be either high or low producers of interferon.

Thus considerable information is available concerning the genetic control of the production of human IFN-β and IFN-α and mouse interferons. In contrast, there is no information to date concerning the genetic control of the production of IFN-γ. When we turn, however, to the genetic control of the *response* to interferon, progress has been made not only for IFN-α and IFN-β, but also for IFN-γ (C. J. Epstein and Epstein, 1982). The interferon response gene mapped in man by the examination of the response of mouse–human somatic cell hybrids to human IFN-α was originally designated *AVP* (for antiviral protein) and now termed *IFRC* (for interferon receptor). It was found on human chromosome 21 (Tan *et al.*, 1973; Slate *et al.*, 1978), which is of particular interest because it is the chromosome which, when present in an extra dose (trisomy 21) gives rise to Down's Syndrome. Later studies refined the localization of the *IFRC* gene to the long arm of chromosome 21 (Tan and Greene, 1976) and, more specifically, to the region from band q 21 to the end of the long arm (Epstein and Epstein, 1976). Using somatic cell hybridization techniques similar to those employed for mapping the human gene, we (Cox *et al.*, 1980; Epstein *et al.*, 1980a) and others (Lin *et al.*, 1980) have also mapped mouse *IFRC* to chromosome 16. The inference that the mouse and human *IFRC* genes actually subsume the same function is greatly strengthened by the findings that two other genes known to be on human chromosome 21, cytoplasmic superoxide dismutase-1 (*SOD*-1) (Franke and Taggart, 1979; Cox *et al.*, 1980; Epstein *et al.*, 1980a; Lin *et al.*, 1980) and phosphoribosyl glycinamide synthetase (*PRGS*) have also been mapped to mouse chromosome 16 (Cox *et al.*, 1981).

Confirmatory studies for the mapping of *IFRC* to chromosome 21 have been based on the analysis of gene dosage effects in diploid and aneuploid human cells. Trisomy 21 (T 21) fibroblasts are more sensitive than diploid cells (matched with regard to tissue and site of origin, genotype if possible, and passage number) to the antiviral effects of IFN-α and IFN-β and monosomy 21 cells are less sensitive (Tan *et al.*, 1974a; Epstein and Epstein, 1976). A similar enhancement of the sensitivity of T 21 cells to interferon has been observed in cells other than fibroblasts and with assays other than antiviral: T 21 fibroblasts are more sensitive to the antiproliferative effect of interferon (Tan, 1976); T 21 peripheral blood monocytes to the anti-maturational effect (Epstein *et al.*, 1980c); stimulated T 21 lymphocytes to the antimitogenic effect (Cupples and Tan, 1977; Gurari-Rotman *et al.*, 1978; Epstein and Epstein, 1980); and T 21 fibroblasts to the reduction of the ratio of 28S to 18S RNA (Maroun, 1979).

An understanding of the mechanism of the greatly enhanced sensitivity of T 21 cells to the effects of interferon must be based on knowledge of the identity of the *IFRC* product. The present consensus is that this product is a cell surface receptor for interferon (Chany *et al.*, 1975), but formal proof of this is still lacking. The major arguments in favour of its being a receptor include the species specific nature of the response being assayed (Creagan *et al.*, 1975) and the inhibition of interferon action by antibodies directed against chromosome 21 determined cell surface constituents (Revel *et al.*, 1976; Slate and Ruddle, 1979b; Kamarck *et al.*, 1981).

We have recently obtained additional evidence consistent with *IFRC* being the gene for the interferon receptor. The expectation for a primary gene dosage response would be that trisomic cells would synthesize 1·5 times as much of the gene product than would diploid cells. If this product were a cell surface receptor which interacted with its ligand according to conventional receptor kinetics, and if the direct intracellular response to binding of the ligand were proportional to the number of receptors occupied, then it would follow that, for any given ligand concentration, trisomic cells would show a 1·5 times greater response than normal cells (L. B. Epstein *et al.*, 1981). In recent studies we used the synthesis of several interferon induced intracellular peptides (demonstrable on autoradiograms of two-dimensional gel electrophoresis) as a measure of this (Weil *et al.*, 1980). First we proved that in the absence of interferon, the pattern of peptides produced by trisomic and normal cells are, with very few exceptions, the same (Weil and Epstein, 1979). We then explored the nature of interferon peptides produced by matched trisomic and diploid fibroblast strains in response to human IFN-α (Weil *et al.*, 1980). We found 12 polypeptides whose concentrations are altered following treatment with IFN-α, 10 of which represent newly induced peptides. Of these, six are of 80 000 daltons, two of 60 000 daltons, one of 40 000 daltons, and one of 37 000 daltons, and all are undetectable in extracts from untreated cells. Two additional polypeptides, with approximate molecular weights of 39 000 and 37 000 daltons were observed in untreated cells, but appeared to undergo an interferon induced interconversion. Using densitometry we found that the relative responses in trisomic and diploid cells correspond closely to expected gene dose relationships over a range of IFN-α concentrations from 0·5 to 5 000 units/ml, with the trisomic cells synthesizing, on the average, about 1·5 times as much of the peptides as did the diploid cells. These data thus provide strong support for the *IFRC* gene product being a surface receptor.

All of the work on *IFRC* described above was carried out with IFN-α or IFN-β, but we have also had a long standing interest in determining whether human chromosome 21 is also involved in the response to human IFN-γ. In our early studies of the sensitivity of T 21 and diploid fibroblasts to the antiviral effects of interferon, we observed the same enhanced sensitivity of the trisomic cells to a crude PHA stimulated IFN-γ preparation as was found with α and β interferons (Epstein and Epstein, 1976). Recently we found the same to be true for a partially purified SEA induced IFN-γ tested on two pairs of matched T 21 and diploid cell strains (L. B. Epstein *et al.*, 1981). It thus appears that human chromosome 21 is involved in the response to IFN-γ, but it is still not known whether the same *IFRC* locus that governs the response to α or β interferons or another chromosome 21 locus is responsible. Additional evidence to support the role of chromosome 21 in governing the response to IFN-γ comes from our recent studies in which we studied the new peptides synthesized in response to IFN-γ (L. B. Epstein *et al.*, 1981). The peptides induced appeared to be the same for IFN-γ and IFN-α, and 1·5–2 times more of the peptides are synthesized in T 21 than in diploid cells. At the present time, we do not know whether IFN-γ, IFN-α, and IFN-β interact with the same receptors. There is disagreement in the literature as to whether the time for development of the antiviral state by IFN-γ is prolonged (Dianzani *et al.*, 1978) or equal to that of IFN-α and β (Falcoff *et al.*, 1980), and it appears that protein synthesis is required for the antiviral action of IFN-γ but not for the other interferons (Dianzani *et al.*, 1980).

The most direct evidence for the actual existence of an interferon receptor is provided by the work of Aguet (1980) who demonstrated the high affinity binding of ^{125}I-labelled purified mouse interferon to cells sensitive to the action of interferon. Apparent saturation of the receptor could be demonstrated, and a significant proportion of the binding was inhibited by unlabelled interferon. L 1210 R cells, which are resistant to the action of interferon demonstrated only a low level of nonspecific binding. Thus it was of particular interest when Hovanessian *et al.* (1980a) demonstrated that the L 1210 R cells were inducible for the $(2'p5'A)_n$ synthetase and protein kinase by IFN-γ, but not, as has been found by other investigators, by IFN-α and IFN-β (Marti *et al.*, 1981).

Also there is evidence that the interferons behave differently with regard to the blocking effect of gangliosides, where the antiviral and antigrowth activities of mouse IFN-β but not of IFN-γ are inhibited (Ankel *et al.*, 1980).

If more than one receptor is involved it remains to be determined whether the same chromosome is responsible or whether each is coded for by a different chromosome.

It is entirely possible, judging from the number of new peptides induced in response to IFN-α and IFN-γ (Hovanessian *et al.*, 1980b; Rubin and Gupta, 1980; Weil *et al.*, 1980; L. B. Epstein *et al.*, 1981) that additional biochemical pathways essential for the action of IFN-α and IFN-γ will be discovered.

There already have been a variety of biochemical responses identified as being induced or enhanced after treatment of cells with interferon. These include the synthesis of specific peptides, as mentioned above, but also the synthesis of specific enzymes [$(2'p5'A)_n$ synthetase and protein kinase] (Hovanessian, 1979). However there are examples in the literature which demonstrate that the IFN-α or IFN-β mediated antiviral state can exist in the absence of these enzymes (Meurs *et al.*, 1981), that the enzyme levels do not always correlate with the degree of antiviral protection (Wood and Hovanessian, 1979; Hovanessian *et al.*, 1981), and that certain cells with constitutively high enzyme levels do not respond to the antiviral effects of interferon (Verhagen *et al.*, 1980). What is important for the purposes of our discussion however is that IFN-γ has also been shown to induce these enzymes (Hovanessian *et al.*, 1980a,b) but there again the induction of the enzymes was not always sufficient for the development of the antiviral or anticellular effects of the IFN-γ (Vandenbussche *et al.*, 1981). Also there has been one report that the kinetics of induction of the $(2'p5'A)_n$ synthetase by IFN-γ is delayed as compared with that of the other interferons and that protein synthesis is required in the former situation, but not in the latter (Baglioni and Maroney, 1980).

VII SUMMARY OF SIMILARITIES AND DIFFERENCES

In trying to summarize all that I have written before in this chapter I shall not make specific reference to the many investigators who have contributed information to each point, as their contributions have been acknowledged in the preceding text.

With regard to the primary structure of IFN-γ nothing is known; the purification, although while well underway, has not been complete enough to allow for determination of amino acid content or terminal amino acid sequence. It does appear from the molecular weight determinations of human IFN-γ, however, that it can exist as a larger molecular weight form than IFN-α and IFN-β with molecular weights in the range of 36 000–58 000 daltons, but also can be in a 20 000 and 25 000 molecular weight form. It is less stable to low pH and heat and has a narrower host range than IFN-α. It also has different antigenic determinants, as it is not neutralized by antisera to human IFN-α or β, but it does have a polynucleotide binding site as do the other interferons. Numerous laboratories throughout the world are currently involved in attempts to purify IFN-γ to homogeneity, to isolate the mRNA for its production, and to clone it by recombinant DNA techniques. Its mRNA has already been translated by several laboratories.

As yet, nothing has been reported as to the genetic control of the production of IFN-γ, but human chromosome 21 has been implicated in the control of its response, both with regard to its antiviral actions and its ability to induce specific new peptides in cells with which it interacts. It is not known whether the genetic locus on chromosome 21 which controls the response to IFN-γ is the same as that which has been regionally mapped for IFN-α and IFN-β to the distal segment of the long arm of the chromosome.

We do not know for certain whether IFN-γ has the same or different receptor(s), or whether its interaction with its receptors occurs in the same or different manner from that of the other interferons. Evidence that suggests a different receptor or a different interaction includes the observation of different rank order of potency of the various interferons depending on the cell type tested, possible differences in the kinetics of induction of antiviral action and induction of specific enzymes, the requirement for protein synthesis for expression of the antiviral effect and induction of specific enzymes by IFN-γ and not by the other interferons, and the ability of IFN-γ to induce specific enzymes in cells that are known to be resistant to the antiviral and enzyme inducing effects of the other interferons. In addition, IFN-γ does not bind to gangliosides, and its antiviral and anticellular effects are not blocked by gangliosides, as is the situation with the other interferons.

Despite all this, however, the same enzymes and peptides can be induced by IFN-γ as by the other interferons. All the interferons also share in common their ultimate actions—the ability to protect cells against viruses and their ability to produce numerous immunoregulatory and other effects on the biology of normal and malignant cells. No unique action or function for IFN-γ has been found to date which distinguishes it as a separate functional entity from the other interferons.

The development of antisera to the various interferons has allowed the characterization of the interferons produced in response to various agents. First, such studies have proved beyond a doubt that a given inducer can induce more than one type of interferon, and second, certain agents which were thought to be exclusively inducers of IFN-γ (i.e. PHA, PPD, *C. parvum*) can also induce IFN-α and another (i.e. Con A), thought also to be exclusively an inducer of IFN-γ, can also induce IFN-β. However, whether the same mechanism of induction obtains for each interferon is not yet known.

The range of cell types producing IFN-γ is more narrow than that which produces the other interferons. IFN-γ is produced by cells of the immune system (i.e. T and B lymphocytes) and the interaction of such cells with macrophages is required for the production of IFN-γ in response to certain inducers, but not to others. However lymphocytes and cells of the monocyte–macrophage lineage are also capable of producing IFN-α. Thus to date, there is no unique or exclusive source of IFN-γ. Cells which produce IFN-γ have the capacity to produce other interferons, but cells, like fibroblasts and epithelial cells which produce both IFN-β and IFN-α have not been found to produce IFN-γ. Once monoclonal antibody to IFN-γ becomes readily available, the nature and proportion of cells producing it in response to a given inducer in normal and disease states can be elucidated.

Finally, let us deal with the issue that has, perhaps, attracted the greatest attention to IFN-γ: its potency. There are examples in the literature in which IFN-γ has been shown to be more potent than the other interferons for its immunoregulatory, antitumour, and antiviral actions and for its ability to transfer resistance to virus across species. In contrast are several equally convincing studies which indicate that its immunoregulatory, antitumour and antiviral effects are less or equipotent to those of IFN-α or IFN-β. All of the studies employed amounts of the various interferons which gave equal antiviral effects on cell types different than those used for testing potency. As various interferons have a various rank order of potency on different cells, it is essential that preparations of equal molarity be used in such comparative studies. At the present time all units used to describe IFN-γ are unique for a given laboratory, and, as such, are arbitrary. They will continue to be arbitrary until an international standard is developed, hopefully in the near future. Precise resolution of the question of relative potency of IFN-γ depends on its purification to homogeneity at which time it can be compared, microgram for microgram, with the other interferons with regard to all their known biologic effects. And, in the final analysis, the question of how IFN-γ is different from IFN-α and IFN-β will really be resolved once its primary, secondary and tertiary structures are elucidated.

VIII PROSPECTS FOR THE FUTURE OF IFN-γ

There are many reasons for continuing work on IFN-γ. On a personal, intellectual and scientific level, if one is interested in the immune system, how it functions, and how the complex series of cellular and molecular interactions occur to result in an immune response and if one is interested in regulation of cell proliferation, then IFN-γ would be very satisfying and rewarding to work with. IFN-γ truly is a "model lymphokine" (Epstein,

1981). It is a product of the immune response and in *in vitro* models it has been shown to influence numerous aspects of the immune response but the underlying mechanism and biochemical events for each of these effects has not yet been worked out. The *in vitro* systems for working with production or action of IFN-γ are well established in the literature and hence are easy to establish and perform in one's own laboratory. The only problem which periodically haunts those of us with conscience who work with *in vitro* models of the immune response is whether the events which we study *in vitro* are relevant to those which occur *in vivo*. After these periodic bursts of frustration and dismay with this issue we return to the security of our tissue culture laboratories safe, sound and secure with the rationalization that we are truly doing "basic research" and that its *in vivo* relevance will undoubtedly be validated in future research.

Not only is IFN-γ of considerable intellectual and scientific interest, but also of tremendous commercial interest as well. This has been demonstrated by the numerous commercial, private, or university based laboratories now devoted to its production in large quantities by conventional or recombinant DNA techniques, its purification and eventual sequencing. The object of many such ventures is to prepare enough IFN-γ for future clinical trials on patients with malignancy or infectious diseases, or in patients with immunological defects. However at present the amount of information available on which these trials would be based is very limited. IFN-γ has been tested *in vivo* against only three murine tumour systems, osteosarcoma (Crane *et al.*, 1978); P 388, a mouse leukaemia induced originally by 3-methylcholanthrene (Fleischmann *et al.*, 1980); and MC 36, a methylcholanthrene induced sarcoma (Salvin *et al.*, 1975). Arguments exist both pro and con for applying the results of studies on the antitumour effects of interferon in animals for consideration of dose, route of administration and duration of therapy in man (Gresser, 1980).

Perhaps more relevant are the results of *in vitro* tests with human tumours. But here too the data are limited. De Ley *et al.* (1980) have reported inhibition of the growth of human lymphoblastoid cells (Daudi and Molt-4) by IFN-γ, but to my knowledge no other work has been published to date. Using an *in vitro* semisolid agar culture system it has been possible to identify human tumours which are sensitive to the antiproliferative effects of IFN-α and IFN-β (Epstein *et al.*, 1980d; Salmon, 1980; Bradley and Ruscetti, 1981), and this technique could well be applied to the study of IFN-γ. Furthermore, in our studies on ovarian carcinoma which employed this technique we found that tumour cells cultured in the presence of cells of the immune system found in ascitic fluid samples were far more sensitive to the antiproliferative effects of IFN-α than were cells derived from solid tumour samples (Epstein *et al.*, 1980e). The explanation for this phenomenon is yet to be determined, but might relate to whether interferon acts directly on the tumour cells or more likely in an indirect manner via its effect on cells of the immune system. Thus future studies with this culture system and other *in vitro* techniques (Sikora *et al.*, 1980) would be of major importance in determining the range of human tumours that respond to the antiproliferative effects of IFN-γ and the other interferons and the nature of the interaction of the interferons with the tumour cells and cells of the immune system. Also, as the semisolid agar culture system has been shown to be predictive of *in vivo* resistance to antitumour drugs with considerable accuracy and also to be predictive of *in vivo* response to a lesser degree (Salmon *et al.*, 1980), it will be important to determine whether similar relationships between *in vitro* and *in vivo* sensitivity also obtain for the various interferons (Epstein and Marcus, 1981). Such information would be of special benefit in screening out patients who would be likely *not* to respond to interferon therapy.

At present, there are only scant data on which to base clinical trials of IFN-γ in infectious diseases, also. IFN-γ does have antiviral protective effects *in vitro* against numerous viruses, some of which in man cause profound illness. For example, IFN-γ generated from mixed murine splenic lymphocyte cultures was shown *in vitro* to protect mouse macrophages against murine hepatitis and influenza viruses (Virelizier *et al.*, 1977); and SEA induced human IFN-γ protected human fibroblasts against vaccinia virus *in vitro* (Rubin and Gupta, 1980). Perhaps more relevant to those events which occur in man infected with a given virus would be the demonstration that IFN-γ has antiviral activity against the virus from which a viral antigen preparation had been made and used to induce the IFN-γ. To my knowledge there is only one report of this nature, and it is with a herpes virus, but in a bovine system (Babiuk and Rouse, 1976).

Thus, there is considerable need for investigators to continue to work with IFN-γ as much information is yet to be learned. Specifically, we need to define:

(1) the primary, secondary, and tertiary structure of IFN-γ and its relationship to the structure and functions of other interferons. Once the structure of IFN-γ is known and the structure is correlated with function, it might be possible to construct an interferon that embodies maximum activity of a given function without becoming immunogenic.

(2) the chromosomes and nucleotide sequence of the genes which control the production of and response to IFN-γ. The ultimate genetic definition of the response to interferon will have to address all of the structural and regulatory components of the response system and provide not only the specific chromosomal locations of the individual genes in the system but also how these genes interact and are regulated;

(3) the biochemistry of the action of IFN-γ.

(4) the mechanism of induction of IFN-γ.

(5) the precise localization (with monoclonal antibodies to IFN-γ) of the proportions and nature of the cell type or types which produce IFN-γ in response to given inducers.

(6) the abnormalities of IFN-γ production in malignancy, infectious disease, immunodeficiency and autoimmunity. Deficiency in IFN-γ production may then be characterized as to whether it is due to an absent or malfunctioning cell population.

(7) the range of antiviral spectrum of IFN-γ *in vitro*, and to determine to what extent IFN-γ is an important part of the host defence mechanisms against a given virus.

(8) the types of human tumours that will respond to IFN-γ *in vitro*, the nature of the interaction of the interferon with the tumour cells or cells of the immune system which express antitumour activity and the nature of the interaction of interferon with other antitumour agents.

The scope of work yet to be done on IFN-γ is mind boggling, but tremendously gratifying in its complexity and challenge.

IX ACKNOWLEDGEMENTS

The experimental results from my laboratory and the work on this chapter were supported by NIH grant CA 27903 and a grant from the National Foundation March of Dimes 6-126.

I wish to thank my mother, Mrs Mary Frances Barth, who sustained me and my family while I worked on this chapter. I also thank my daughter, Joanna Epstein, who had nothing but the best of wishes for my rapid progress, Mary Evelyn Rose for her patience, encouragement and skill in typing the manuscript, and Mary Lou Sumberg for skillful editorial assistance.

X REFERENCES

Aguet, M. (1980). *Nature, Lond.* **284**, 459–461.

Allen, G. and Fantes, K. H. (1980). *Nature, Lond.* **287**, 408–411.

Ankel, H., Krishnamurti, C., Besancon, F., Stefanos, S. and Falcoff, E. (1980). *Proc. natn. Acad. Sci. U.S.A.* **77**, 2528–2532.

Archer, D. L., Smith, B. G., Ulrich, J. T. and Johnson, H. M. (1979). *Cell. Immun.* **48**, 420–426.

Babiuk, L. A. and Rouse, B. T. (1976). *Infect. Immun.* **13**, 1567–1578.

Baglioni, C. and Maroney, P. A. (1980). *J. biol. Chem.* **255**, 8390–8393.

Baron, S., Brunnell, P. A. and Grossberg, S. E. (1979). *In* "Antiviral Agents and Viral Diseases of Man" (eds G. Galasso, T. C. Merigan, and R. A. Buchanan), pp. 151–208. Raven, New York.

Beck, J., Engler, H., Brunner, H. and Kirchner, H. (1980). *J. Immun. Meth.* **39**, 63–73.

Berg, K. and Heron, J. (1980). *Scand. J. Immun.* **11**, 489–502.
Blalock, J. E., Georgiades, G. A. and Johnson, H. M. (1979). *J. Immun.* **122**, 1018–1021.
Blalock, J. E., Georgiades, J. A., Langford, M. P., and Johnson, H. M. (1980). *Cell. Immun.* **49**, 390–394.
Bourgeade, M. F., Chany, C. and Merigan, T. C. (1980). *J. gen. Virol.* **46**, 449–454.
Bourgeade, M. F., Rousset, S., Paulin, D. and Chany, C. (1981). *J. Interferon Res.* **1**, 323–332.
Bradley, E. C. and Ruscetti, F. W. (1981). *Cancer Res.* **41**, 244–249.
Bryson, Y. L., Winter, H. S., Gard, S. E., Fischer, T. J. and Stiehm, E. R. (1980). *Cell. Immun.* **55**, 191–200.
Burke, D. C. (1980). *In* "Interferon 1980" (ed. I. Gresser) pp. 47–64. Academic Press, London and New York.
Burke, D. C. and Meager, A. (1980). *Ann. N.Y. Acad. Sci.* **350**, 179–187.
Chang, T. W., Testa, D., Kung, P. C. and Goldstein, G. (1981). *Fedn Proc. Fedn Am. Socs exp. Biol.* **40**, 1048.
Chany, C. (1981). *Lymphokine Rep.*, in press.
Chany, C., Vignal, M., Couillin, P., Van Cong, N., Boue, J. *et al.*, (1975). *Proc. natn. Acad. Sci. U.S.A.* **72**, 3129–3134.
Cox, D. R., Epstein, L. B. and Epstein, C. J. (1980). *Proc. natn. Acad. Sci. U.S.A.* **77**, 2168–2172.
Cox, D. R., Goldblatt, D. and Epstein, C. J. (1981). *Am. J. hum. Genet.*, **33**, 145A.
Crane, J. L., Glasgow, L. A., Kern, E., and Youngner, J. S. (1978). *J. natn. Cancer Inst.* **61**, 871–874.
Creagan, R. P., Tan, Y. H., Chen, S. and Ruddle, F. H. (1975). *Fedn Proc. Fedn Am. Socs exp. Biol.* **34**, 2222–2226.
Cupples, C. G. and Tan, Y. H. (1977). *Nature, Lond.* **267**, 165–167.
de Ley, M., van Damme, J., Claeys, H., Weening, H., Heine, J. W. *et al.* (1980). *Eur. J. Immun.* **10**, 877–883.
De Maeyer, E. and De Maeyer-Guignard, J. (1979). *In* "Interferon 1979" (ed. I. Gresser), pp. 75–100. Academic Press, London and New York.
De Maeyer-Guignard, J., Thang, M. N. and De Maeyer, E. (1977). *Proc. natn. Acad. Sci.* **74**, 3787–3790.
De Maeyer-Guignard, J., Tovey, M., Gresser, I., and De Maeyer, E. (1978). *Nature, Lond.* **271**, 622–625.
Derynck, R., Content, J., De Clercq, E., Volckaert, G., Tavernier, J. *et al.* (1980a). *Nature, Lond.* **285**, 542–547.
Derynck, R., Remaut, E., Saman, E., Stanssens, P., De Clercq, E., Content, J. and Fiers, W. (1980b). *Nature, Lond.* **287**, 193–197.
Dianzani, F., Salter, L., Fleischmann, W. R. Jr, and Zucca, M. (1978). *Proc. Soc. exp. Biol. Med.* **159**, 94–97.
Dianzani, F., Zucca, M., Scupham, A. and Georgiades, J. A. (1980). *Nature, Lond.* **283**, 400–402.
Djeu, J., Timonen, T. and Herberman, R. B. (1981). *Immunobiology* **159**, 85.
Epstein, C. J. and Epstein, L. B. (1982). *Tex. Rep. Biol. Med.*, in press.
Epstein, C. J., Epstein, L. B., Cox, D. R. and Weil, J. (1981). *In* "Trisomy 21. An International Symposium" (eds G. R. Burgio, M. Fraccaro, L. Tiepolo and U. Wolf), pp. 155–172. Springer-Verlag, Berlin.
Epstein, L. B. (1977). *In* "Interferons and their Actions" (ed. W. E. Stewart II) pp. 91–132. CRC Press, Cleveland, Ohio.
Epstein, L. B. (1978). *Tex. Rep. Biol. Med.* **35**, 43–56.

Epstein, L. B. (1979). *In* "Biology of the Lymphokines" (eds. S. Cohen, E. Pick, and J. J. Oppenheim) pp. 443–514. Academic Press, New York.
Epstein, L. B. (1981). *Fedn Proc. Fedn Am. Socs exp. Biol.* **40**, 56–61.
Epstein, L. B. (1982). *Tex. Rep. Biol. Med.*, in press.
Epstein, L. B. and Ammann, A. J. (1974). *J. Immun.* **112**, 617–626.
Epstein, L. B. and Cline, M. J. (1974). *Clin. Exp. Immun.* **16**, 553–563.
Epstein, L. B. and Epstein, C. J. (1976). *J. infect. Dis.* **133**, Suppl. A56–A62.
Epstein, L. B. and Epstein, C. J. (1980). *Cell. Immun.* **51**, 303–318.
Epstein, L. B. and Gupta, S. (1981). *J. clin. Immun.*, **1**, 186–194.
Epstein, L. B. and Marcus, S. (1981). *Cancer Chem. Pharm.*, in press.
Epstein, L. B. and Smith, C. W. (1968). *J. Immun.* **100**, 421–435.
Epstein, L. B. and Stohlman, F., Jr (1964). *Blood*, **24**, 69–75.
Epstein, L. B., Cline, M. J. and Merigan, T. C. (1971a). *J. clin. Invest.* **50**, 744–753.
Epstein, L. B., Cline, M. J. and Merigan, T. C. (1971b). *Cell. Immun.* **2**, 602–613.
Epstein, L. B., Stevens, D. A. and Merigan, T. C. (1972). *Proc. natn. Acad. Sci. U.S.A.* **69**, 2632–2636.
Epstein, L. B., Kreth, H. W. and Herzenberg, L. A. (1974). *Cell. Immun.* **12**, 407–421.
Epstein, L. B., Cox, D. R. and Epstein, C. J. (1980a). *Ann. N.Y. Acad. Sci.* **350**, 171–173.
Epstein, L. B., Goldblatt, D., Yu, K., Dean, J., Herberman, R. B. *et al.* (1980b). *In* "Biochemical Characterization of Lymphokines" (eds A. De Weck, F. Kristensen and M. Landy) pp. 353–358. Academic Press, New York.
Epstein, L. B., Lee, S. H. S. and Epstein, C. J. (1980c). *Cell Immun.* **50**, 191–194.
Epstein, L. B., Shen, J. T., Abele, J. S. and Reese, C. C. (1980d). *Ann. N.Y. Acad. Sci.* **350**, 228–244.
Epstein, L. B., Shen, J. T., Abele, J. S., and Reese, C. C. (1980e). *In* "Cloning of Human Tumor Cells" (ed. S. Salmon) pp. 277–290. Alan Liss, New York.
Epstein, L. B. Weil, J., Lucas, D. O., Cox, D. R. and Epstein, C. J. (1981). *In* "The Biology of the Interferon System" (eds E. De Maeyer, G. Galasso, and H. Schellekens), pp. 247–256. Elsevier/North Holland, Amsterdam.
Falcoff, E., Weitzerbin, J., Stefanos, S., Lucero, M., Billardon, C. and Catinot, L. (1980). *Ann. N.Y. Acad. Sci.* **350**, 145–156.
Farrar, W. L., Johnson, H. M. and Farrar, J. J. (1981). *J. Immun.* **126**, 1120–1125.
Fleischmann, W. R., Jr, Georgiades, J. A., Osborne, L. C. and Johnson, H. M. (1979). *Infect. Immun.* **26**, 248–253.
Fleischmann, W. R., Jr, Kleyn, K. M. and Baron, S. (1980). *J. Natn. Cancer Inst.* **65**, 963–966.
Francke, U. and Taggart, R. T. (1979). *Proc. natn. Acad. Sci. U.S.A.* **76**, 5230–5233.
Friedman, R. M. and Cooper, H. L. (1967). *Proc. Soc. exp. Biol. Med.* **125**, 901–905.
Fujisawa, J., Iwakura, Y., and Kawade, Y. (1978). *J. biol. Chem.* **253**, 8677–8679.
Georgiades, J. A., Langford, M. L., Stanton, G. J. and Johnson, H. M. (1979). *IRCS Med Sci.* **7**, 559.
Goeddel, D. V., Shepard, H. M., Yelverton, E., Leung, B. and Crea, R. *et al.* (1980a). *Nucleic Acids Res.* **8**, 4057–4074.
Goeddel, D. V., Yelverton, E., Ullrich, A., Heyneker, H. L., Miozzari, G. *et al.* (1980b). *Nature, Lond.* **287**, 411–416.
Goeddel, D. V., Leung, D. W., Dull, T. J., Gross, M., Lawn, R. M. *et al.* (1981). *Nature, Lond.* **290**, 20–25.

Goldstein, L. D., Georgiades, J. A., Langford, M. P., Stanton, G. J. and Johnson, H. M. (1979). *IRCS Med. Sci.* **7**, 560.

Green, J. H., Cooperband, S. R. and Kibrick, S. (1969). *Science, N.Y.* **164**, 1415–1417.

Gresser, I. (1980). *Recent Results Cancer Ther.* **75**, 226–228.

Gresser, I. and Bourali, C. (1970). *J. natn. Cancer Inst.* **45**, 365–376.

Gresser, I., De Maeyer-Guignard, J., Tovey, M. G. and De Maeyer, E. (1979). *Proc. natn. Acad. Sci. U.S.A.* **76**, 5308–5312.

Gurari-Rotman, D., Revel, M., Tartakovsky, B., Segal, S., Hahn, T. *et al.* (1978). *FEBS Lett.* **94**, 187–190.

Havell, E. A. and Carter, W. A. (1981). *Virology* **108**, 80–86.

Hayes, T. G., Yip, Y. K. and Vilcek, J. (1979). *Virology* **98**, 351–363.

Heine, J. W., de Ley, M., Van Damme, J., Billiau, A. and De Somer, P. (1980). *Ann. N.Y. Acad. Sci.* **350**, 364–373.

Herberman, R. B. (Ed.) (1980). "Natural Cell Mediated Immunity against Tumors." Academic Press, New York.

Hochkeppel, H. K., Menge, U. and Collins, J. (1981). *Nature, Lond.* **291**, 500–501.

Houghton, M., Eaton, M. A. W., Stewart, A. G., Smith, J. C., Doel, S. M. *et al.* (1980). *Nucleic Acids Res.* **8**, 2885–2893.

Hovanessian, A. G. (1979). *Differentiation* **15**, 139–151.

Hovanessian, A. G., La Bonnardiere, C. and Falcoff, E. (1980a). *J. Interferon Res.* **1**, 125–135.

Hovanessian, A. G., Meurs, E., Aujean, O., Vaquero, C., Stefanos, S. *et al.* (1980b). *Virology* **104**, 195–204.

Hovanessian, A. G., Meurs, E. and Montagnier, L. (1981). *J. Interferon Res.* **1**, 179–190.

Isaacs, A. and Lindenmann, J. (1957). *Proc. R. Soc. Lond.* **147**, 258–267.

Isaacs, A., Lindenmann, J. and Valentine, R. C. (1957). *Proc. R. Soc. Lond.* B **147**, 268–273.

Ito, Y., Nishiyama, Y., Shimokata, K., Takeyama, H. and Kunii, A. (1979). *Microbiol. Immun.* **23**, 1169–1177.

Ito, Y., Aoki, H., Kimura, Y., Takano, M., Maeno, K. *et al.* (1980). *Infect. Immun.* **28**, 542–545.

Ito, Y., Aoki, H., Kimura, Y., Takano, M., Shimokata, K. *et al.* (1981). *Infect. Immun.* **31**, 519–523.

Iwakura, Y., Yonehara, S. and Kawade, Y. (1978). *J. biol. Chem.* **253**, 5074–5079.

Jameson, P. and Grossberg, S. E. (1979). *Arch. Virol.* **62**, 209–219.

Johnson, H. M., Stanton, G. J. and Baron, S. (1977). *Proc. Soc. exp. Biol. Med.* **154**, 138–141.

Karmack, M. E., Slate, D. L., D'Eustachia, P., Barel, B. and Ruddle, F. H. (1981). *Fedn Proc. Fedn Am. Socs exp. Biol.* **40**, 1051.

Kawakita, M., Cabrer, B., Taura, H., Rebello, M., Slattery, E., Weideli, H. and Lengyel, P. (1978). *J. biol. Chem.* **253**, 598–602.

Kirchner, H., Zawatsky, R., Engler, H., Schirrmacher, V., Becker, H. *et al.* (1979). *Eur. J. Immun.* **9**, 824–826.

Kirchner, H., Fenkel, H., Zawatsky, R., Engler, H. and Becker, H. (1980). *Eur. J. Immun.* **10**, 224–225.

Knight, E., Jr (1976). *Proc. natn. Acad. Sci. U.S.A.* **73**, 520–523.

Knight, E., Jr (1980). *In* "Interferon 1980" (ed. I. Gresser) pp. 1–12. Academic Press, London and New York.

Knight, E., Jr, Hunkapiller, M. W., Korant, B. D., Hardy, R. W. F., and Hood, L. E. (1980). *Science, N.Y.* **207**, 525–526.

Koistinen, V. and Cantell, K. (1981). Report presented at a meeting in Warwick, England.

Kraft, D., Rumpold, H., Steiner, R., Radaszkiewicz, T. and Swetly, P. (1981). *Immunobiology* **159**, 137.

Landolfo, S., Kirchner, H., and Simon, M. M. (1981). *Immunobiology* **159**, 88.

Langford, M. P., Weigent, D. A., Georgiades, J. A., Johnson, H. M. and Stanton, G. J. (1981). *J. Immun.* **126**,, 1620–1623.

Lawn, R. M., Adelman, J., Dull, T. J., Gross, M., Goeddel, D. *et al.* (1981). Science, N.Y. **212**, 1159–1162.

Lee, S. H. S., Lee, C. L. Y. and Rozee, K. R. (1981). *Can. Soc. Microbiol.* Abstracts of Annual Meeting, Abstract E8, 101.

Levy, W. P., Shively, J., Rubinstein, M., Del Valle, U., and Pestka, S. (1980). *Proc. natn. Acad. Sci. U.S.A.* **77**, 5102–5104.

Lin, P. F., Slate, D. L., Lawyer, F. C. and Ruddle, F. H. (1980). *Science, N.Y.* **209**, 285–287.

Lipinski, M., Virelizier, J. L., Tursz, T. and Griscelli, C. (1980). *Eur. J. Immun.* **10**, 246–249.

Lucas, D. O. and Epstein, L. B. (1981). *In* "Physiology of the Reticulo-endothelial System: A Comprehensive Treatise" (eds S. M. Reichard and J. P. Filikins). Vol. 4. Plenum. New York. In press.

Lucero, M. A., Weitzerbin, J., Stefanos, D., Billardon, C., Falcoff, E. *et al.* (1980). *Cell. Immun.* **54**, 58–69.

Maeda, S., McCandliss, R., Gross, M., Sloma, A., Familletti, P. C. *et al.* (1980). *Proc. natn. Acad. Sci. U.S.A.* **77**, 7010–7013.

Marcucci, F., Waller, M., Kirchner, H. and Krammer, P. (1981). *Nature, Lond.* **291**, 79–81.

Maroun, L. E. (1979). *Biochem. J.* **179**, 221–225.

Marti, J., Vandenbussche, P., Silhol, M., Milhaud, P., Verhaegen, M. *et al.* (1981). *J. Interferon Res.* **1**, 287–295.

Masucci, M. G., Zigetti, R., Klein, E., Klein, G., Gruest, J. *et al.* (1980). *Science, N.Y.* **209**, 1431–1435.

Meager, A., Graves, H., Burke, D. C., and Swallow, D. M. (1979). *Nature, Lond.* **280**, 493–495.

Meurs, E., Hovanessian, A. G. and Montagnier, L. (1981). *J. Interferon Res.* **1**, 219–232.

Mizrahi, A., O'Malley, J. A., Carter, W. A., Takasuki, A., Tamura, G. *et al.* (1978). *J. biol. Chem.* **253**, 7612–7615.

Morgan, M. J. and Faik, P. (1977). *Br. J. Cancer* **35**, 254.

Nagata, S., Taira, H., Hall, A., Johnsrud, L., Streuli, M., Ecsodi, J., Boll, W., Cantell, K. and Weissmann, C. (1980a). *Nature, Lond.* **284**, 316–320.

Nagata, S., Mantei, N. and Weissmann, C. (1980b). *Nature, Lond.* **287**, 401–408.

Nagata, S., Brack, C., Henco, K., Schambock, A. and Weissmann, C. (1981). *J. Interferon Res.* **1**, 333–336.

Ortaldo, J. R., Alvarez, J. M. and Timonen, T. (1981). *Immunobiology* **159**, 139.

Osborne, L. C., Georgiades, J. A. and Johnson, H. M. (1979). *Infect. Immun.* **23**, 80–86.

Osborne, L. C., Georgiades, J. A. and Johnson, H. M. (1980). *Cell. Immun.* **53**, 65–70.

Owerbach, D., Rutter, W. J., Shows, T. B., Gray, P., Goeddel, D. V. *et al.* (1981). *Proc. natn. Acad. Sci. U.S.A.* **78**, 3123–3127.

Pang, R. H. L., Hayes, T. G. and Vilček, J. (1980). *Proc. natn. Acad. Sci.* **77**, 5341–5345.

Perussia, B., Mangoni, L., Engers, H. D. and Trinchieri, G. (1980). *J. Immun.* **125**, 1589–1595.

Peter, H. H., Dallügge, H., Zawatsky, R., Euler, S., Leibold, W. *et al.* (1980). *Eur. J. Immun.* **10**, 547–555.

Pfeffer, L. M., Wang, E. and Tamm, I. (1980). *J. cell. Biol.* **85**, 9–17.

Ratcliff, T. C., McCool, R. E. and Catalona, W. J. (1981). *Cell. Immun.* **57**, 1–12.

Revel, M., Bash, D. and Ruddle, F. H. (1976). *Nature, Lond.* **260**, 139–141.

Roberts, N. J., Jr, Douglas, R. G., Simons, R. M. and Diamond, M. E. (1979). *J. Immun.* **123**, 365–369.

Rubin, B. Y. and Gupta, S. L. (1980). *Proc. natn. Acad. Sci. U.S.A.* **77**, 5928–5932.

Rubinstein, M., Rubinstein, S., Familletti, P. C., Miller, R. S., Waldman, A. A. and Pestka, S. (1979). *Proc. natn. Acad. Sci. U.S.A.* **76**, 640–644.

Salmon, S. E. (1980). *In* "Cloning of Human Tumor Stem Cells" (ed. S. E. Salmon) pp. 291–314. Alan Liss, New York.

Salmon, S. E., Alberts, D. S., Meyskens, F. L., Durie, B. G. M., Jones, S. E. *et al.* (1980). *In* "Cloning of Human Tumor Stem Cells" (ed. S. E. Salmon) pp. 223–246. Alan Liss, New York.

Salvin, S. B., Youngner, J. S., Nishio, J. and Neta, R. (1975). *J. Natn. Cancer Inst.* **55**, 1233–1235.

Sato, T. and Yaname, I. (1981). *In Vitro* **17**, 244, Abstract 181.

Secher, D. S. (1981). *Nature, Lond.* **290**, 501–503.

Secher, D. S. and Burke, D. C. (1980). *Nature, Lond.* **285**, 446–450.

Sehgal, P. (1981). *Antiviral Res.* Abstract 1, 4.

Sehgal, P. B. and Sagar, A. D. (1980). *Nature, Lond.* **288**, 95–97.

Senik, A., Stefanos, S., Kolb, J. P., Lucero, M. and Falcoff, E. (1980). *Ann. Immun.* **131**C, 349–361.

Shoham, J., Eshel, I., Aboud, M. and Salzberg, S. (1980). *J. Immun.* **125**, 54–58.

Sikora, K., Basham, T. Dilley, J., Levy, R. and Merigan, T. (1980). *Lancet,* **ii**, 891–893.

Slate, D. L. and Ruddle, F. H. (1979a). *Cell* **16**, 171–180.

Slate, D. L. and Ruddle, F. H. (1979b). *Pharm. Ther.* **4**, 221–230.

Slate, D. L. and Ruddle, F. H. (1980). *Ann. N.Y. Acad. Sci.* **350**, 174–178.

Slate, D. L., Shulman, L., Lawrence, J. B., Revel, M. and Ruddle, F. H. (1978). *J. Virol.* **25**, 319–325.

Sonnenfeld, G. (1980). *Lymphokine Rep.* **1**, 113–131.

Sonnenfeld, G., Mandel, A. D. and Merigan, T. C. (1977). *Cell Immun.* **34**, 193–206.

Staehlin, T., Durrer, B., Schmidt, J., Takacs, B., Stocker, J. *et al.* (1981). *Proc. natn. Acad. Sci. U.S.A.* **78**, 1848–1852.

Stanwick, T. L., Campbell, D. E. and Nahmias, A. J. (1981). *Immunobiology* **158**, 207–212.

Starr, S. E., Dalton, B., Garrabrant, T., Paucker, K. and Plotkin, S. A. (1981). Infect. Immun. **30**, 17–22.

Stefanos, S., Catinot, L., Wietzerbin, J., and Falcoff, E. (1980). *J. gen. Virol.* **50**, 225–229.

Stewart, W. E. II (1979). "The Interferon System." Springer, Wien, New York.

Stewart, W. E., II *et al.* (1981). *J. Interferon Res.* **1**, v–vi.

Streuli, M., Nagata, S. and Weissmann, C. (1980). *Science, N.Y.* **209**, 1343-1347.
Sugiyama, M. and Epstein, L. B. (1978). *Cancer Res.* **38**, 4467-4473.
Taira, H., Broeze, R. J., Jayaram, B. M., Lengyel, P., Hunkapiller, M. W. and Hood, L. E. (1980). *Science, N.Y.* **207**, 528-530.
Tan, Y. H. (1976). *Nature, Lond.* **260**, 141-142.
Tan, Y. H. (1977). *In* "Interferons and Their Actions" (ed. W. E. Stewart II) pp 73-90. CRC Press, Cleveland, Ohio.
Tan, Y. H. and Greene, A. E. (1976). *J. gen. Virol.* **32**, 153-157.
Tan, Y. H., Tischfield, J. and Ruddle, F. H. (1973). *J. exp. Med.* **137**, 317-330.
Tan, Y. H., Creagan, R. P. and Ruddle, F. H. (1974a). *Proc. natn. Acad. Sci. U.S.A.* **71**, 2251-2255.
Tan, Y. H., Schneider, E. L., Tischfield, J., Epstein, C. J. and Ruddle, F. H. (1974b). *Science, N.Y.* **186**, 61-63.
Tan, Y. H., Barakat, F., Berthold, W., Smith-Johannsen, H. and Tan, C. (1979). *J. biol. Chem.* **254**, 8067-8073.
Tanaka, Y., Epstein, L. B., Brecher, G. and Stohlman, F., Jr (1963). *Blood* **22**, 614-629.
Taniguchi, T., Ohno, S., Fujii-Kuriyama, Y. and Muramatsu, M. (1980a). *Gene* **10**, 11-15.
Taniguchi, T., Guarente, L., Roberts, T. M., Kimelman, D., Douhan, J. and Ptashne, M. (1980b). *Proc. natn. Acad. Sci. U.S.A.* **77**, 5230-5233.
Taniguchi, T., Pang, R. H. L., Yip, Y. K., Henriksen, D. and Vilček, J. (1981). *Proc. natn. Acad. Sci. U.S.A.* **78**, 3469-3472.
Taylor-Papadimitriou, J. (1980). *In* "Interferon 1980" (ed. I. Gresser) pp. 13-46. Academic Press, London and New York.
Timonen, T., Saksela, E., Virtanen, I. and Cantell, K. (1980). *Eur. J. Immun.* **10**, 422-427.
Trinchieri, G., Perussia, B. and Santoli, D. (1980). *In* "Natural Cell Mediated Immunity Against Tumors" (ed. R. Herberman) pp. 655-670. Academic Press, New York.
Ullrich, A., Dull, T. J., Gray, A. and Lawn, R. M. (1981). *Science, N.Y.* **212**, 1159-1162.
Vandenbussche, P., Divizia, M., Verhaegen-Lewalle, M., Fuse, A., Kuwata, T. *et al.* (1981). *Virology* **111**, 11-22.
Verhagen, M., Divizia, M., Vandenbussche, P., Kuwata, T. and Content, J. (1980). *Proc. natn. Acad. Sci. U.S.A.* **77**, 4479-4483.
Vilček, J., Havell, G. A. and Yamazaki, S. (1977). *Ann. N.Y. Acad. Sci.* **284**, 703-710.
Vilček, J., Sulea, I. T., Volvovitz, F., and Yip, Y. K. (1980). *In* "Biochemical Characterization of Lymphokines" (eds A. de Weck, F. Kristensen, and M. Landy) pp. 323-330. Academic Press, New York.
Virelizier, J. L., Allison, A. C. and De Maeyer, E. (1977). *Infect. Immun.* **17**, 282-285.
Virelizier, J. L., Lenoir, G. and Griscelli, C. (1978). *Lancet* **ii**, 231-234.
Wallace, D. M., Hitchcock, M. J. M., Reber, S. B. and Berger, S. (1981). *Biochem. biophys. Res. Commun.* **100**, 865-871.
Weigent, D. A., Langford, M. P., Smith, E. M., Blalock, J. E. and Stanton, G. J. (1981). *Infect Immun.* **32**, 508-512.
Weil, J. and Epstein, C. J. (1979). *Am. J. hum. Genet.* **31**, 478-488.
Weil, J., Epstein, L. B. and Epstein, C. J. (1980). *J. Interferon Res.* **1**, 111-124.
Wheelock, E. F. (1965). *Science, N.Y.* **149**, 310-311.

Wietzerbin, J., Stefanos, S., Falcoff, R., Lucero, M., Catinot, L. *et al.* (1978a). *Infect. Immun.* **21**, 966–972.
Wietzerbin, J., Stefanos, S., Lucero, M. and Falcoff, E. (1978b). *Biochem. biophys. Res. Commun.* **85**, 480–489.
Wietzerbin, J., Stefanos, S., Lucero, M., Falcoff, E., O'Malley, J. *et al.* (1979). *J. gen. Virol.* **44**, 773–781.
Wiranowska-Stewart, M. (1981). *J. Interferon Res.* **1**, 315–321.
Wiranowska-Stewart, M. and Stewart, W. E., II (1981). *J. Interferon Res.* **1**, 233–244.
Wiranowska-Stewart, M., Lin, L., Braude, I. A. and Stewart, W. E., II (1980). *Mol. Immun.* **17**, 625–633.
Wood, J. N. and Hovanessian, A. G. (1979). *Nature, Lond.* **282**, 74–76.
Wussow, P. V., Platsoucas, C. D., Wiranowska-Stewart, M. and Stewart, W. E. II (1981). *Immunobiology* **159**, 84.
Yip, Y. K., Pang, R. H. L., Urban, C. and Vilček, J. (1981). *Proc. natn. Acad. Sci. U.S.A.* **78**, 1601–1605.
Zoon, K. C., Smith, M. E., Bridgen, P. J., Zur Nedden, D., and Anfinsen, C. B. (1979). *Proc. natn. Acad. Sci. U.S.A.* **76**, 5601–5605.
Zoon, K. C., Smith, M. E., Bridgen, P. J., Anfinsen, C. B., Hunkapiller, M. W. and Hood, L. E. (1980). *Science, N.Y.* **207**, 527–528.

Interferon and Natural Killer Cells

EERO SAKSELA

Department of Pathology, University of Helsinki, Finland

I INTRODUCTION

Natural killer cells (NK cells) are characterized by their ability to mount a rapid cytotoxic response against tumour derived or virus infected target cells without known prior sensitization or intentional immunization. They were originally discovered in *in vitro* cytotoxicity tests where tumour patients' cell mediated immunity against cultured cancer cells was measured and compared to control persons' similar activity. The latter exhibited various levels of spontaneous cytotoxicity, which was first discarded as "background noise" but since the recognition of the NK system underlying the phenomenon (Takasugi *et al.*, 1973) an avalanche of research activity has ensued (for reviews see Möller, 1979; Herberman, 1980). By various cell fractionation studies it could be established that the effector cells did not belong in the categories of conventional T cells, B cells or monocyte–macrophages and they were thus designated natural killer (NK) cells. The interest has been mainly stimulated by the notion that NK cells may potentially form an effective first-line defence against tumour cells arising within the organism. The NK cell system seems to possess a considerable degree of autonomous regulatory capacity, in which interferon plays a crucial role. As interferon has shown promise in tumour control in its own right (Gresser, 1977) it is perhaps not surprising that a great deal of interest has been focused on the mechanisms by which interferon controls the NK system.

II NK CELLS AND TUMOUR RESISTANCE

The *in vivo* data suggesting a role for NK cells in tumour resistance stem from mouse studies, and indirect findings pointing to the same direction are also emerging in man. These studies have been recently reviewed (Herberman and Holden, 1978; Roder and Haliotis, 1981) and will not be touched upon in further detail. Here I have compiled in Table I the main lines of evidence associating NK cells with tumour cell surveillance and control as a background for the discussion of the role of interferon as a regulator of the NK system.

TABLE I *In vivo* correlations suggesting a role of NK cells in tumour surveillance

1.	Correlation of high NK activity and tumour transplant resistance in genetic crosses of inbred mouse strains
2.	Resistance of thymus-less nude mice (which have an increased NK activity) to NK sensitive tumour cells and their normal incidence of spontaneous tumours
3.	Murine lymphocytes enriched for NK cells and depleted of other cell types inhibit NK sensitive tumour growth when transferred at the time of tumour challenge
4.	The NK status of the bone marrow donor determines the NK activity and resistance to NK sensitive tumours of irradiated and bone marrow-reconstituted recipients
5.	NK deficient beige mutant mice have an impaired resistance against NK sensitive tumours and their metastases
6.	Tumour promoters inhibit and retinoic acid augments murine NK cell activity
7.	Carcinogens depress murine NK cell activity
8.	NK deficient Chediak-Higashi patients develop a "lymphoma-like accelerated phase"
9.	Lymphoma patients already at early clinical stages have an impaired NK activity
10.	Immunodeficient patients and immunosuppressed kidney graft recipients have low NK activity and high incidence of malignancy

III EFFECT OF INTERFERON ON NK CELL ACTIVITY

The basic findings associating interferon with the NK system were the observations that interferon could boost NK cell activity in mice (Gidlund *et al.*, 1978; Herberman *et al.*, 1979). Administration of interferon subcutaneously or intraperitoneally into mice increased the spontaneous NK mediated cytotoxicity of peritoneal exudate, spleen and blood cells against NK sensitive targets. Interferon itself was the mediator since the same effect could be obtained with preparations purified to electrophoretic homogeneity and anti-interferon antiserum could inhibit the boosting effect.

Various interferon inducers, such as polyinosinic–polycytidylic acid (poly I–C), *Corynebacterium parvum*, bacille Calmette-Guérin (BCG) and pyran copolymer also stimulate NK activity in mice. This effect is apparently dependent on macrophages since various treatments impairing the macrophage function prevent the boosting of NK activity (Djeu *et al.*, 1979b). Interferon is, however, the mediator of the augmentation since the effect is inhibited by anti-interferon antiserum (Djeu *et al.*, 1979a) and mice which are congenitally poor responders to interferon induction do not show the NK boosting effect (Örn *et al.*, 1981). If such mice are irradiated and reconstituted with bone marrow grafts from good responders, the capacity to react with augmented NK activity to the various interferon inducers is also restored (Haller *et al.*, 1977). It is important to note that the route of administration of the inducers seems to play a crucial role in the type of response elicited. When *corynebacterium parvum* was given intraperitoneally a good boosting effect of the NK activity was seen, whereas intravenous administration resulted in a depression of the NK killing capacity of both spleen and peritoneal exudate derived effector cells (Ojo *et al.*, 1978). The findings thus suggested the existence of yet other controlling pathways of the NK activity, differentially affected by interferon inducing agents, which depended on the route of administration (discussed later in this review).

The interferon-mediated boosting of NK activity has been demonstrated also in other experimental animals and in man. Treatment of human peripheral blood-derived effector cells with interferon increases their cytolytic activity several fold (Einhorn *et al.*, 1978). Depending on the initial level of activity the increase in terms of lytic units may be 5–8-fold and the minimum dose required for the effect is between 10 and 100 IU/ml of interferon. The effect is an all-or-none type of response—further increase of the dose of interferon does not increase the cytotoxic activity. The effector cells may be pretreated with interferon and washed prior to addition on the target cells, and in this case less than five minutes' pretreatment is enough to give a full response. The augmentation is sensitive to actinomycin and puromycin indicating a need for RNA and protein synthesis (Ortaldo *et al.*, 1980). The interferon-boosted cytotoxic activity is also blocked by monensin, indicating that it is mediated by similar cellular secretion associated pathways as that of interferon nontreated NK cells (Carpén *et al.*, 1981a). All types of interferon are active in augmenting the NK cytolysis. α interferons derived from leukocytes, lymphoblastoid cell lines or *E. coli*, β interferon obtained from fibroblasts as well as γ interferon have been shown to exert this effect.

Healthy volunteers as well as tumour patients receiving interferon injections respond with an increased level of NK activity in the blood (Einhorn, 1980). The intramuscular or subcutaneous injections of interferon (usually 3×10^6 IU daily) are followed by an augmented NK activity in the blood reaching its maximum within 24 h. During the first 4–6 h there is in most cases an initial drop of NK activity (Kariniemi *et al.*, 1980), which seems to coincide with the temperature rise associated with injections of semipurified as well as highly purified preparations of interferon. An augmented level of NK activity is maintained during the interferon treatment, but the activity returns to original levels after cessation of the injections (Einhorn, 1980; Huddlestone *et al.*, 1979).

It is difficult to say what role the increased NK activity plays in the effects of interferon on the clinical outcome of malignant disease. Many investigators have failed to find NK activity among the mononuclear cells infiltrating human solid tumours although the blood levels of NK activity are within normal range (Klein *et al*, 1980; Tötterman *et al.*, 1978). We have investigated three patients with untreated ovarian carcinoma, who received 3×10^6 units of interferon 18 h prior to operation, in order to examine whether interferon might induce invasion of NK cells into the tumour tissue. An increased blood NK activity was seen following the interferon injection but no cytotoxic activity among the tumour-infiltrating cells. It is possible that circulating, potentially metastatic cells are more effectively eliminated by the interferon augmented NK cells (Hanna and Fidler, 1980). At least it is known that human neoplasms do contain target structures rendering them susceptible to NK lysis (Vanky *et al.*, 1981).

IV INTERFERON INDUCTION AT TARGET CELL CONTACT

Another basic observation that led to the recognition of the intimate association of interferon and NK activity was the finding that interferon synthesis was induced in human leukocytes brought into contact with established, mainly tumour-derived, tissue culture cell lines (Trinchieri *et al.*, 1978). It was conclusively shown that the interferon-producing cells were leukocytes, not the cultured cells which acted as inducers. Simultaneously with the interferon release the NK activity of the leukocyte populations was greatly enhanced, and the mediator of the enhanced activity was shown to be interferon (Trinchieri and Santoli, 1978). Thus, for instance, cells such as fetal fibroblasts that are unable to induce interferon did not enhance the NK activity of co-cultured leukocytes, and addition of anti-interferon serum into the co-cultures of inducing cells and leukocytes inhibited the augmentation of NK activity.

Later, it has been shown that also a chronic virus-carrier state can render originally non-inducing tissue culture cells to good promoters of leukocyte interferon synthesis (Minato *et al.*, 1980). The interferon produced at the contact of leukocytes with established, mainly tumour-derived cell lines or with chronically virus-infected cells is of the pH 2 resistant leukocyte interferon (α-IFN) type. Whether small amounts of γ-interferon are also simultaneously produced has not been established. The latter point is interesting in view of the findings that interferon is produced in mixed leukocyte cultures of lymphocytes stemming from histo-incompatible individuals (Baron *et al.*, 1980; Perussia *et al.*, 1980). In this system the interferon released in the supernatants is of the γ-interferon, "immune interferon" type. As mentioned above, γ interferon is also an efficient enhancer of NK activity and apparently plays a role in the induction of the "anomalous" cytotoxicity, generated rapidly during the first days of mixed leukocyte cultures (Seeley and Golub, 1978). This cytotoxicity has the characteristic nonspecificity of NK mediated cytolysis in contrast to the antigen-specific killing created later in the same cultures and mediated by cytotoxic T cells.

The exact relationship of the "malignant" nature or virus-carrier state of the inducing cells to their interferon inducing capacity has not been clarified in detail. The lack of full knowledge of the structures on target-cell surfaces involved in the induction and in the cytolytic pathway of NK cells makes final judgement on this question impossible. Suggestions have been made that the inducing capacity would be dependent on mycoplasma contamination acquired during *in vitro* culture of the established cell lines used as inducers (Beck *et al.*, 1980). This is made unlikely by the findings of several authors that the most sensitive methods of detection involving fluorochrome staining of mycoplasma DNA have not been able to show such a contamination in the inducing cells. It is also noteworthy that tumour cells dispersed directly from human solid primary neoplasms are able to induce interferon in short-term co-incubations with leukocytes (Tarkkanen *et al.*, 1981). It is thus more likely that the interferon-inducing capacity is related to the cell surface changes associated with the neoplastic or viral carrier state.

V NATURE OF THE INTERFERON-PRODUCING CELL

For understanding of the regulatory mechanisms leading to activation of the NK mediated cytotoxicity it is important to ascertain which leukocyte subpopulation harbours the producer cells of interferon or whether this is a more or less general property of various blood cell types. In simple fractionation steps of blood leukocytes, the granulocytes have been eliminated as potential producer cells (see Epstein, 1979). Removal of the adherent monocyte-macrophages improves the cell-induced interferon producing capacity and no interferon can be induced by cell contact from the adherent cells themselves. Fractionation of the remaining, adherent cell-depleted leukocyte populations on discontinuous gradients of Percoll (Pharmacia, Sweden) resulted in an enrichment of the interferon-producing capacity in fractions consisting of 75–85% of large lymphocytes with characteristic azurophilic granules in their relatively abundant cytoplasm (Timonen *et al.*, 1980). Such large granular lymphocytes (LGLs) have been shown to be the mediators of human NK activity and consequently also in the fractionations above, the NK activity and interferon-producing capacity peaked at the same lymphocyte fractions. In addition to LGL these fractions contained medium-sized and small lymphocytes (almost exclusively T cells) and some monocytes. With indirect immunofluorescence using either "polyvalent" sheep anti-interferon serum or monoclonal antibodies it could be shown that of these cell types only the LGL had demonstrable interferon in the cytoplasm (Fig. 1) following induction with erythroleukaemia (K-562) cells (Timonen *et al.*, 1980; Saksela *et al.*, 1981).

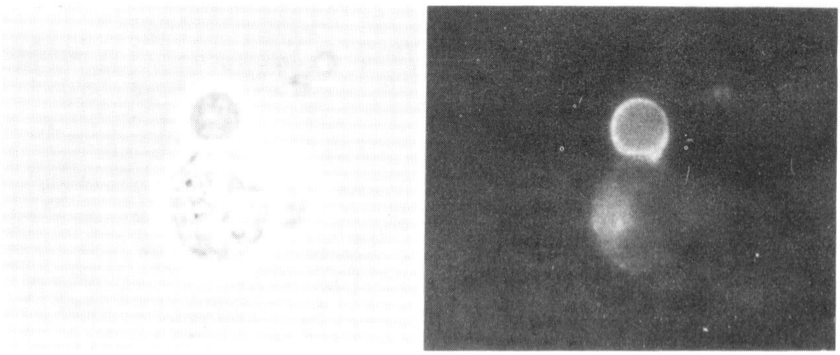

Fig. 1 Indirect immunofluorescence using monoclonal anti α interferon antiserum (courtesy of Dr D. Secher, MRC Laboratory of Molecular Biology, Cambridge, England) on human NK cells of large granular lymphocyte (LGL) type allowed to be in contact with interferon-inducing K-562 erythroleukaemia cells for 6 h. Note bright cytoplasmic fluorescence on LGL cells (arrow).

Thus, LGLs were the producers of interferon at target cell contact and as the same population also harboured the NK cytolytic activity it appeared that the NK cell itself was responsible for the production.

Large granular lymphocytes share characteristics of both the T lymphocyte and monocyte-macrophage lineages. However, there are important differences which make the assignment of a specific lineage difficult at present. For instance, LGLs do not react with the monoclonal OKT-3 antisera which is considered to be a pan T marker, and enzymologically as well as in their surface glycoprotein pattern LGLs are distinct from monocyte-macrophages (Ortaldo *et al.*, 1981; Saksela and Timonen, 1980). It is quite possible that they represent an independent lineage which in man constitutes about 3% of all leukocytes (10–15% of lymphocytes). LGL-type cells are also responsible for the NK activity in most of the other species studied with the notable exception of mice whose NK activity resides in small lymphocytic cells without distinctive morphological features (Roder *et al.*, 1978). Functionally, LGLs are nonphagocytic, nonadherent cells which carry receptors for the Fc portion of IgG. Through their Fc receptors LGLs are efficient mediators of antibody dependent cellular cytotoxicity (ADCC) and may, in fact, be the main mediators of this activity (Timonen *et al.*, 1981a). Also, in mice the NK cells have been suggested to be the principal effector cells in ADCC (Ojo and Wigzell, 1978). It is noteworthy that interferon effectively stimulates the ADCC activity of blood and spleen leukocytes, further substantiating the contention that both NK and ADCC activities reside in the same or largely overlapping population of cells.

VI FEEDBACK REGULATION OF THE NK ACTIVITY

As the data reviewed above implicated human NK cells themselves as the producers of interferon at tumour target contact, two possible mechanisms of the augmentation of NK activity by interferon could be visualized. Either interferon increased the cytolytic activity of each individual effector cell or it increased the number of active cells. The *in vivo* evidence obtained in rodents favoured the latter interpretation. Oehler and Herberman (1978) showed that irradiation and treatment with various immunopharmacological drugs depleted the NK active cells from rat peritoneal cavity. However, interferon could rapidly restore the activity apparently by recruiting originally noncytolytic cells into cytotoxic activity. The recovery of the NK activity occurred within hours after interferon induction indicating that cell proliferation was not involved, and pre-existent inactive "pre-NK" cells were apparently turned on by interferon. In the human system we could demonstrate a similar phenomenon by using target cell adsorption elution techniques. In experiments where cells were allowed to attach on fetal fibroblasts, which do not induce interferon production, and separated from nonattaching cells, we could show that interferon treatment did not increase the NK activity of the fibroblast binding cells which we termed "mature" NK cells. In contrast, the cell population depleted of "mature" NK cells by fibroblast adsorption and showing a greatly diminished NK activity became strongly NK cytotoxic by interferon treatment (Saksela *et al.*, 1979a). It thus appeared that the human "pre-NK" cells had a lower avidity for fetal fibroblast targets and were not bound in the adsorption experiments. These cells were able to rapidly turn on their cytotoxic activity in response to interferon treatment.

The analysis of the morphology of the attacker cells in effector/target conjugates of interferon activated "pre-NK" cells showed that they had also a typical LGL morphology (Timonen *et al.*, 1979). So far we have not been able to find markers that would allow other than functional separation of the "mature" and "pre-NK" cells. Recent experiments with single effector/single target conjugate assays have substantiated the conclusion that the augmentation of human NK activity occurs predominantly via recruitment of an originally noncytolytic "pre-NK" pool into full cytotoxic activity rather than via an increase of the cytotoxic potential of each individual NK cell (Targan and Dorey, 1980; Silva *et al.*, 1980). Experiments in mice have shown that this mechanism also operates there. Mouse NK cells carry a surface marker, Ly 5, and treatment of the spleen cell populations with antiserum against Ly 5 plus complement removes the NK activity. However, subsequent treatment with interferon restores the NK activity, which is again susceptible to abrogation by anti Ly 5 and complement (Minato *et al.*, 1980). Interferon thus recruits a "pre-NK" population into cytotoxic activity and simultaneously induces the expression of the "mature" NK marker antigen on the surface of the cells.

The above techniques allowed also a further dissection of the interferon-producing cells within the NK cell system. The fetal fibroblast-binding cells were separated from the nonbinding cells and both populations were allowed to stay in contact with interferon-inducing K-562 erythroleukaemia cells. Good titres of interferon were obtained in the supernatants of fibroblast binding "mature" NK/K-562 co-cultures whereas the nonbinding, "pre-NK" containing populations were poor interferon producers (Timonen *et al.*, 1980). Similarly, in mice, the interferon-producing cells at inducing cell contact were sensitive to treatment with anti Ly 5 serum plus complement (Minato *et al.*, 1980). Thus, both in man and mice the "mature" NK cells seemed to be the prime producers of interferon when stimulated with suitable target cells. On the basis of these findings a positive feedback type of amplification loop could be conceived as operating within the NK system itself, with interferon as a mediator, as depicted in Fig. 2.

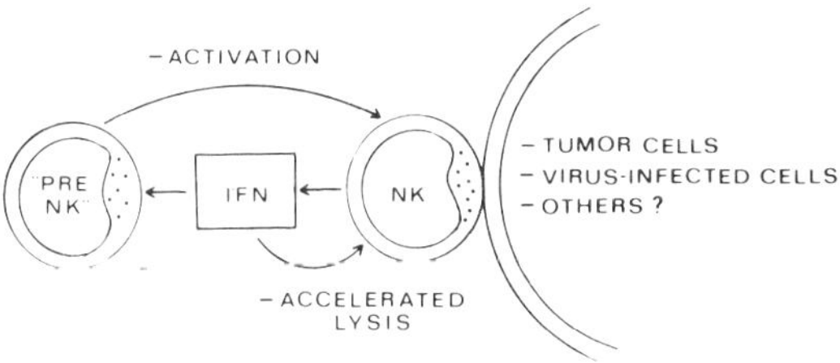

Fig. 2 Positive feedback regulation of NK activity through interferon.

This model implies that "mature" circulating NK cells are highly avid binders to target cells and release at the contact interferon, which in turn activates "pre-NK" cells into full cytotoxic activity. It is not known whether the interferon activated "pre-NK" cells also acquire the capacity to produce interferon and further amplify the response. The interferon involved in this positive feedback amplification loop of NK activity is of the α interferon type but it is not known which or how many of the α interferon gene products are involved. In single effector/target conjugate assays it has been demonstrated that also "pre-NK" cells are able to bind to highly susceptible NK target cells (Targan and Dorey, 1980; Timonen *et al.*, 1981a). Such target cells apparently carry NK target "receptors" with higher avidity than fetal fibroblasts. The analysis of the time dependence curves of increasing NK mediated cytolysis in conjugates of highly susceptible target cells and NK cells has shown, furthermore, that interferon accelerates the kinetics of lysis and that some activation of the target bound "pre-NK" cells may also occur (Targan and Dorey, 1980). Whether the latter takes place via induction of interferon and subsequent augmentation of the NK activity of the interferon producing cell itself is not known. In these single conjugate assays it has also been shown that the augmented NK cells return to their original level of activity within 6 h and they can be again boosted by a second interferon pulse (Targan and Dorey, 1980).

VII INTERFERON AND NK SUPPRESSOR CELLS

There is accumulating evidence suggesting that the NK system both in man and in experimental animals can be regulated through suppressor cells (see Cudkowicz and Hochman, 1979). Suppressor cells for NK activity have been detected in infant mice (Savary and Lotzova, 1978) and in mice treated with a variety of agents (see Cudkowicz and Hochman, 1979). Adherent, apparently monocyte-macrophage type cells have been implicated in the NK suppression and the effect seems to be mediated by soluble factors released into the supernatants of the suppressor cells (Santoni *et al.*, 1980). In man, adherent cells with suppressive capacity on human NK cells have been found among cells of ovarian carcinoma-induced ascites (Mantovani *et al.*, 1980). It seems, therefore quite established that monocyte-macrophages can inhibit the cytotoxic activity of NK cells.

As indicated above the suppressive activity seems to be mediated by soluble factors and some recent evidence suggests that prostaglandins may be the active molecules (Brunda *et al.*, 1980). It is known that prostaglandins are secreted by activated macrophages (see Keller, 1980). Since interferon can enhance phagocytosis and other capacities of macrophages and via this mechanism presumably also lead to prostaglandin synthesis one could postulate that under some conditions interferon could lead to suppression of the NK activity. This has not been formally shown but some of the interferon injection trials on normal volunteers lend support to this type of response occurring in some situations. As mentioned above, intradermal or intramuscular injection of 3×10^6 IU of interferon is followed by a transient drop of blood NK activity at 4–6 h *post* injection and this drop is accompanied by a practically total disappearance of LGL type cells from the blood (Kariniemi *et al.*, 1980). The drop in NK activity coincides with the maximal fever response. As prostaglandins are known to be involved in fever responses this could be taken as one example where interferon-induced prostaglandin release might be causing a suppression of the NK activity. There are also reports suggesting that inhibition of the prostaglandin synthesis, e.g. by aspirin, may lead to an increased blood NK activity (Droller *et al.*, 1979). Many infectious agents, tissue degradation products and bacterial endotoxins are known to activate macrophages. If macrophage activation is associated with prostaglandin synthesis the ensuing NK suppression could conceivably create possibilities for survival and spread of processes normally controlled by NK cells. Whether such a mechanism may play a role, for instance in certain associations of chronic inflammation and neoplasia, is an intriguing possibility. This pathway could, however, be also potentially important in shutting off the NK lysis and act as a negative feedback link in the regulation of NK activity (see Fig. 3).

Monocyte-macrophages are not the only cells of the lymphoreticular system implicated in the regulation of the NK activity. Circulating small T lymphocytes representing a particular subpopulation characterized by receptors for the Fc portion of IgG, the $T._G$ cells, have also been shown to effectively suppress the cytotoxic activity of enriched human LGL cells (Tarkkanen and Saksela, 1981). The $T._G$ population has been previously shown to contain suppressor cells for other, both antigen-specific and nonspecific T cell functions (see Moretta and Cooper, 1980). The best source for the $T._G$ suppressors of human NK activity was the umbilical cord

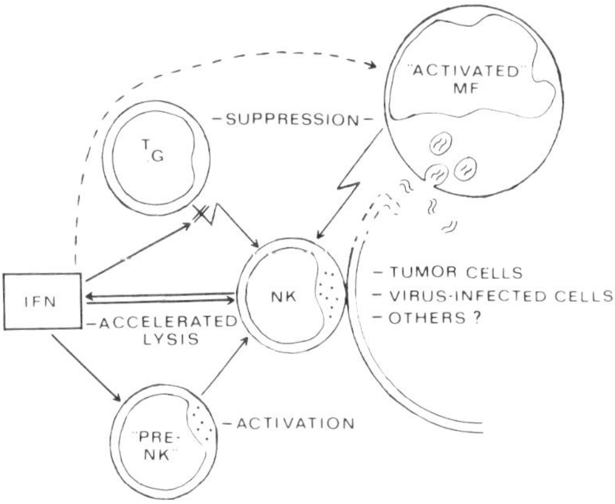

Fig. 3 Possible regulatory pathways of the NK activity involving augmenting and suppressing cellular interactions. Interferons induced at the target cell contact augments the activity by recruiting "pre-NK" cells as shown in Fig. 2 and/or by inhibiting suppressor T cells. Note that macrophages activated by tissue degradation products of lysed cells or by other means could potentially act as a negative feedback link.

blood, where these cells circulated apparently in higher numbers or in a higher state of activity than in adult peripheral blood. Their easier demonstrability in the umbilical cord blood may be related to a physiological need to suppress histo-incompatibility-related responses in the feto-maternal relationship. It is known that in histo-incompatible mixed leukocyte cultures NK activity is rapidly enhanced as mentioned above, and suppression of this activity may be important to prevent tissue damage in the fetus. The $T._G$ population has been shown to contain also suppressor cells inhibiting the maternal PHA and Con-A-induced lymphocyte blastogenesis (Olding and Oldstone, 1974; Oldstone and Tishon, 1977). Whether the suppressive effects are mediated by the same or different subpopulations of $T._G$ cells is not known. Suppressor $T._G$ cells capable of inhibiting the human NK activity have also been isolated from the blood of patients with untreated laryngeal and kidney carcinomas as well as from nor normal blood donors (Tarkkanen, unpublished data) but strictly quantitative comparisons are still lacking.

Interferon inhibits the activity of the human NK $T._G$ suppressor cells. Pretreatment of the $T._G$ suppressor cells with interferon for an hour prior to addition on the NK effectors completely abrogates the suppressive capacity of the cells (Tarkkanen and Saksela, 1981). This mechanism forms thus an additional possible pathway of increasing the NK activity by interferon. As, however, most of the increased NK activity after interferon administration seems to be related to the recruitment of "pre-NK" cells into full cytotoxic activity the role of this suppressor inhibition pathway remains to be elucidated. As the preparations of interferon used in the *in vitro* experiments are mixtures of numerous interferon gene products, the various pathways of regulation outlined above and schematically depicted in Fig. 3 may be preferentially operating with certain types of interferon under *in vitro* conditions and under physiological dose ranges.

VIII OTHER NK REGULATORY EFFECTS OF INTERFERON

In the foregoing, the effects of interferon on the NK effector and regulatory cells have been considered. However, interferon may also interact with the target cells and alter their responses to the cytolytic activity of NK cells. Trinchieri and Santoli (1978) showed that pretreatment of target cells with interferon alters their susceptibility to NK cell-mediated lysis and, in particular, normal cells such as diploid fibroblasts are subject to this modulation. It has been postulated that the protective effect of interferon on normal cells in contrast to virus-infected cells or tumour cells would be an important mechanism in directing the cytotoxic activity of NK cells in a teleologically sensible fashion. In later experiments some tumour-derived cells have also been shown to be protected by interferon (Welsh *et al.*, 1981) and it has been demonstrated that the net cytotoxic result is a balance of the target-protecting and NK-stimulating effects of interferon (Moore *et al.*, 1980). In the bone marrow derived, NK sensitive physiological target cell model discussed in detail later, interferon does seem to have a similar protective role (Hansson and Kiessling, 1981). The protection seems to be related to the expression of interferon receptors on the target cell surface. Thus, primitive F-9 teratocarcinoma cells not expressing interferon receptors could not be protected whereas more differentiated teratocarcinoma lines with interferon receptors showed good protection (Welsh *et al.*, 1981).

Suggestions have also been made that contact of the NK cells with sensitive targets leads to a certain degree of inactivation of the effector cells making them unable to continue the cytolytic activity (Trinchieri *et al.*, 1978). This phenomenon can be demonstrated only with cells unable to induce interferon synthesis. Treatment of the effector cells with interferon reverses the target cell contact-induced inactivation allowing each individual NK cell to make several lethal hits on subsequent targets. As normal cells seem incapable of inducing interferon synthesis this pathway of NK cell inactivation might also contribute to the exclusion of normal cells from cytolytic damage.

IX "NORMAL" NK TARGETS AND INTERFERON

Some possible mechanisms by which normal cells are exempted from the NK cell mediated cytolytic damage have been shortly touched upon above. However, in the mouse system low levels of NK killing have been shown against syngeneic normal bone marrow cells, macrophages and thymocytes (Nunn *et al.*, 1977). On the other hand, interferon activated NK cells kill a wide array of normal cells (Welsh, 1978). Because of the ubiquitous presence in mouse cells of C-type viruses, which may potentially activate the NK cells via the interferon induction pathway, the mouse data may not unequivocally answer the question of susceptibility of normal tissues to NK cytolytic activity. In man, diploid fetal fibroblasts are relatively sensitive to human NK cytotoxicity (Saksela *et al.*, 1979a). However, in autologous experiments with cultured adult skin fibroblasts as targets, the donor's own blood NK cells, either nonfractionated or enriched into a considerable degree, fail to kill, whereas allogeneic skin fibroblasts are killed (Tarkkanen *et al.*, 1980). When the effector cells are activated by interferon both autologous and allogeneic skin fibroblasts are killed without preference and as efficiently as fetal fibroblasts. Autologous and allogeneic fibroblasts bind LGL-type effector cells equally well and the bound cells function equally well against sensitive third party targets such as K-562 erythroleukaemia cells. It would therefore appear that the circulating "mature" NK cells are somehow suppressed in their autologous cytotoxic ability, whereas the *in vitro* (and possibly *in vivo?*) activated "pre-NK" cells kill without discrimination.

The situation is somewhat different when normal haematopoietic tissues are used as targets. As already mentioned parental bone marrow graft rejection in F-1 hybrid mice is apparently mediated by NK cells and this has led to an important development of the haematopoietic target cell model by Kiessling and his co-workers (see Hansson and Kiessling, 1981). A NK-sensitive, normally occurring target cell population was originally found in the fetal thymus in mice. The occurrence of the sensitive cells was inversely correlated with the NK cell activity of the animal when followed as a function of age (Hansson *et al.*, 1979). Similar NK sensitive target cells have been recently found in human fetal thymus and bone marrow. Such cells are also found in adult bone marrow although the level of sensitivity to NK lysis is considerably lower. These bone marrow target cells are killed without preference and to the same degree by autologous and allogeneic NK effector cells, which have the characteristic LGL morphology described above (Hansson and Kiessling, 1981). Interferon effectively augments the NK cytolysis in this system (Hansson *et al.*, 1981). The inverse reciprocity of the occurrence of NK sensitive targets and NK-active effector cells seen in mouse thymus has also been demonstrated by experiments showing that the adult bone marrow contains NK effectors against the standard K-562 target whereas the fetal bone marrow is completely without NK cytolytic activity. The NK-sensitive targets in the bone marrow seem to be myelomonocytic colony-forming cells since the colony formation in agar is inhibited by the NK active cells in the above combinations (Hansson and Kiessling, 1981). These authors have therefore suggested that NK cells are involved in the regulation of the haemopoietic stem cell proliferation and interferon appears to be an important regulator of this system. It will be of considerable interest to see whether stem cells in other organ systems might also form a natural target cell population for NK cells.

X SOME CHALLENGING *IN VIVO* CORRELATIONS

It should be evident from the foregoing chapters that interferon is involved in a variety of ways in the regulation of the NK system. It will take some time before the true significance of this complicated network in various physiological cell interactions and in disease can be unravelled. Another dimension to the system may be expected to emerge from studies on the relative role of various types of interferon when pure preparations representing the products of the different interferon genes become available, due to the rapid biotechnological development in this area. Interferons seem to represent a family of biologically highly active molecules which may have preferentially weighted roles in the various cellular interactions under physiological conditions. In this respect the results of Virelizier *et al.* (1979) are quite illustrative. These authors found a group of patients with immunological disorders who had a deficient NK activity combined with lacking γ interferon production when tested *in vitro*. Administration of 10^5 IU α interferon intramuscularly restored the NK cell activity indicating that the NK cell system itself was functioning properly. The suggestion, therefore, was that γ interferon which was deficiently produced by these patients was crucial in maintaining the physiological level of NK activity. The recruitment of the "pre-NK" cells could perhaps be visualized as an emergency response activated via α interferon(s) under pathological conditions when aberrant cell variants arise within the organism or when viral or other microbial invasion has occurred.

Another aspect not yet settled in spite of the extensive characterization of the NK cells concerns the possible target subspecificities within the NK system. A case in point is the so-called natural cytotoxic (NC) system in mice which shares most of its characteristics with the NK systems but shows some definite differences possibly related to such target cell subspecificities (Stutman, 1980). The NC cell activity is normal in beige mice which, as already mentioned, are grossly defective in their NK activity (Roder and Duwe, 1979; Stutman and Cuttito, 1981). The lymphoma-like, NK sensitive tumours grow better and metastasize earlier in beige mice than in normal controls (Kärre *et al.*, 1980; Talmadge *et al.*, 1980). However, beige mice show an apparently normal incidence of carcinogen induced solid tumours, and their normal resistance may be related to the normally functioning NC system (Argov *et al.*, 1981). The basic difference between the NK and NC systems is that the former is measured conventionally with YAC or Molt lymphoma target cells in short-term (4 h) assays whereas the latter is measured with anchorage dependent, solid tumour-derived target cells in long-term (18 h) assays. This trivial-sounding technical difference has, however, obvious *in vivo* relevance in the mouse. In man, the bone marrow target model clearly measures the "classical" NK activity commonly assayed with K-562 erythroleukaemia target cells. It may be significant that the only clear relationship between a defective NK activity, as measured in this way, and malignancy has been detected in lymphoma patients (Tursz, 1981). The NK defective patients with Chediak-Higashi syndrome or with X-linked lymphoproliferative syndrome also develop lymphomas or lymphoma-like lesions (see Roder *et al.*, 1981). Whether the long-term assays utilizing anchorage dependent, solid tissue-derived target cells will give further information on similar associations between the incidence of solid tumours and NK activity remains to be seen. The effector cells against both anchorage dependent and independent targets reside in the large granular lymphocyte (LGL) fraction which could contain subpopulations with different target cell preferences perhaps related to their various physiological stem cell targets.

A rather direct demonstration of the power of interferon-augmented natural defence mechanisms *in vivo* has been recently published by Reid *et al.* (1981). These authors showed that a certain tumour-derived cell line regularly produced tumours in nude mice. However, when a chronic virus-carrier state was induced in the tumour cells, nude mice were able to resist tumour cell inoculations and no growth ensued. If the recipient nude mice were simultaneously treated with anti-interferon serum even the virus-infected inoculum cells caused tumour growth. Apparently the virus-carrier state resulted in interferon induction and activation of the NK system which could inhibit tumour growth, and this resistance could be broken by anti-interferon serum.

Some mechanisms which could be effective in protecting normal cells from the NK mediated attack were briefly reviewed above. NK cells have been implicated in various auto-immune diseases which could result from failures at a number of different points of this protective network. An obvious mechanism potentially triggering a NK-mediated attack towards normal constituents is suggested by the findings of interferonaemia in patients with systemic lupus erythromatosus (SLE), rheumatoid arthritis, dermatomyositis and scleroderma (Hooks *et al.*, 1980). It is conceivable that the interferon-mediated inhibition of the suppressor $T_{\cdot G}$ cell function or direct activation of the "pre-NK" cells could form the basis of the tissue damage in these conditions. There are also animal models relevant to this line of argumentation. Gresser and his collaborators (1980) could induce a disease characterized by growth inhibition, liver necrosis and death in newborn mice and rats with high doses of interferon. Shorter treatment resulted in a glomerulonephritis resembling lupus nephritis. When newborn, these rodents have a very low spontaneous NK cell activity, but it can be effectively boosted with interferon. If stem cells are particularly sensitive to the action of NK cells and are poorly protected by interferon due to immaturity and lack of expression of interferon receptors as discussed above, this syndrome could well be mediated by the interferon activated NK system. Further, the auto-immune disease in New Zealand black mice, which is a model of human SLE, can be accelerated by the administration of interferon (Heremans *et al.*, 1978). Auto-immune disease may, therefore, prove to be an important *in vivo* area where aberrations in the finely balanced interferon–NK cell system are involved.

NK cells may be the only cells responding with interferon production to contact with persistently virus-infected cells and the subsequent activation of the cytotoxic NK system can be critical in the elimination of such cells. In multiple sclerosis, a significantly impaired interferon-producing ability of the blood lymphocytes has been described (Minato *et al.*, 1980). As this disease has been considered as one of the prime examples of potentially "slow-virus" induced diseases in man, the possible pathogenetic mechanism outlined above might conceivably contribute to a deficient capacity to eliminate the persistently infected cells and allow slow progression of the disease (Bloom, 1980).

XI CONCLUDING REMARKS

Interferon is intimately involved in the regulation of the NK system. As it seems to be simultaneously a product and a regulator of activity of the NK cells and even affects the level of NK sensitivity of the target cells, a functionally rather flexible semi-autonomous control system is created. The NK system could perhaps be viewed as an ontogenically old homoeostatic system with less refined modes of operation than the highly sophisticated vertebrate immune system. Interferon production is also a highly conserved property of cells throughout the Animal Kingdom. It may have evolved as a protective device at single cell level and later adapted as a messenger and regulator when a "second generation" defensive system evolved in a more complex cellular society. This network of interactions of the interferon-NK system has presumably been endowed with considerable survival power and we are apparently only just beginning to understand the mechanisms of fine tuning within the system and their significance in normal physiology and disease.

XII ACKNOWLEDGEMENTS

Supported by grant No. CA 23809 from the National Institutes for Health, NCI, Bethesda MD, USA. I am grateful to Prof. Kari Cantell, Central Public Health Laboratory, Helsinki, for critical reading of the manuscript.

XIII REFERENCES

Argov, S., Cochran, A. J., Kärre, K., Klein, G. O. and Klein, G. (1981). *Int. J. Cancer.* In press.

Baron, S., Blalock, J. E., Dianzani, F., Fleischmann, W. R., Georgiades Jr, J. A., Johnson, H. M. and Stanton, G. J. (1980). *Ann. N.Y. Acad. Sci.* **350**, 130.

Beck, J., Engler, H., Brunner, H. and Kirchner, H. (1980). *J. Immunol. Methods* **38**, 63.

Bloom, B. R. (1980). *Nature, Lond.* **284**, 593.

Brunda, M. J., Herberman, R. B. and Holden, H. T. (1980). *J. Immun.* **124**, 2682.

Carpén, O., Virtanen, I. and Saksela, E. (1981a). *Cell. Immun.* **58**, 97.

Carpén, O., Virtanen, I. and Saksela, E. (1981b). *J. Immun.* In press.

Cudkowicz, G. and Hochman, P. S. (1979). *Immun. Rev.* **44**, 13.

Djeu, J. Y., Heinbaugh, J. A., Holden, H. T. and Herberman, R. B. (1979a). *J. Immun.* **122**, 175.

Djeu, J. Y., Heinbaugh, J. A., Holden, H. T. and Herberman, R. B. (1979b). *J. Immun.* **122**, 182.

Droller, M. J., Perlman, P. and Schneider, M. V. (1979). *Cell. Immun.* **39**, 154.

Einhorn, S. (1980). *In* "Natural Cell-mediated Immunity Against Tumors" (Ed. R. B. Herberman) p. 529. Academic Press, New York.

Einhorn, S., Blomgren, H. and Strander, H. (1978). *Int. J. Cancer* **22**, 405.

Epstein, L. B. (1979). *In* "Biology of the Lymphokines" (Eds S. Cohen, E. Pick and J. J. Oppenheim) p. 443. Academic Press, New York.

Gidlund, M., Örn, A., Wigzell, H., Senik, A. and Gresser, I. (1978). *Nature, Lond.* **273**, 759.

Gresser, I. (1977). *In* "Cancer—A Comprehensive Treatise" (Ed. F. Becker) pp. 5, 521. Plenum Press, New York.

Gresser, I., Morel-Maroger, L., Riviére, Y., Guillon, J-C. and Tovey, M. G. (1980). *Ann. N.Y. Acad. Sci.* **350**, 12.

Haller, O., Kiessling, R., Örn, A. and Wigzell, H. (1977). *J. exp. Med.* **145**, 1411.

Hanna, N. and Fidler, I. J. (1980). *J. natn. Cancer Inst.* **65**, 801.

Hansson, M. and Kiessling, R. (1981). *In* "NK cells: Fundamental Aspects and Role in Cancer" (Eds R. B. Herberman, C. Rosenfeld and B. Serrou). Human Cancer Immunology, Vol. 6. North-Holland, Amsterdam.

Hansson, M., Kiessling, R., Andersson, B. Kärre, K. and Roder, J. (1979). *Nature, Lond.* **278**, 174.

Hansson, M., Kiessling, R. and Andersson, B. (1981). *Eur. J. Immun.* **11**, 8.

Herberman, R. B. (Ed.) (1980). "Natural Cell-Mediated Immunity Against Tumors". Academic Press, New York.

Herberman, R. B. and Holden, H. T. (1978). *Adv. Cancer Res.* **27**, 305.

Herberman, R. B., Ortaldo, J. R. and Bonnard, G. D. (1979). *Nature, Lond.* **277**, 221.

Heremans, H., Billian, A., Colombatti, A., Hilgers, J. and de Somer, P. (1978). *Infect. Immun.* **21**, 925.

Hooks, J. J., Moutsopoulos, H. M. and Notkins, A. L. (1980). *Ann. N.Y. Acad. Sci.* **350**, 21.

Huddlestone, J. R., Merigan, T. C. and Oldstone, M. B. A. (1979). *Nature, Lond.* **282**, 417.

Kariniemi, A. L., Timonen, T. and Kousa, M. (1980). *Scand. J. Immun.* **12**, 37.

Kärre, K., Klein, G. O., Kiessling, R., Klein, G. and Roder, J. C. (1980). *Nature, Lond.* **284**, 624.

Keller, R. (1980). *In* "Natural Cell-mediated Immunity Against Tumors" (Ed. R. B. Herberman) p. 1219. Academic Press, New York.

Klein, E., Masucci, M. G., Masucci, G. and Vanky, F. (1980). *In* "Natural Cell-mediated Immunity Against Tumors" (Ed. R. B. Herberman) p. 909. Academic Press, New York.

Mantovani, A., Allavena, P., Sessa, C., Bolis, G. and Mangioni, C. (1980). *Int. J. Cancer* **25**, 573.

Minato, N., Reid, L., Neighbour, A., Bloom, B. R. and Holland, J. (1980). *Ann. N.Y. Acad. Sci.* **350**, 42.

Moore, M., White, W. J. and Potter, M. R. (1980). *Int. J. Cancer* **25**, 565.

Möller (Ed.) (1979). Natural killer cells. *Immun. Rev.* **44**.

Moretta, L. and Cooper, M. D. (1980). *In* "Clinical Immunobiology" (Eds F. H. Bach and R. A. Good) p. 4. Academic Press, New York.

Nunn, M. E., Herberman, R. B. and Holden, H. T. (1977). *Int. J. Cancer* **20**, 381.

Oehler, J. R. and Herberman, R. B. (1978). *Int. J. Cancer* **21**, 221.

Ojo, E. and Wigzell, H. (1978). *Scand. J. Immun.* **7**, 297.

Ojo, E., Haller, O., Kimura, A. and Wigzell, H. (1978). *Int. J. Cancer* **21**, 444.

Olding, L. B. and Oldstone, M. B. A. (1974). *Nature, Lond.* **249**, 161.

Oldstone, M. B. A. and Tishon, A. (1977). *Nature, Lond.* **269**, 333.

Örn, A., Gidlund, M., Wigzell, H. and Gresser, I. (1981). *Eur. J. Immun.* In press.

Ortaldo, J. R., Phillips, W., Wasserman, K. and Herberman, R. B. (1980). *J. Immun.* **125**, 1839.

Ortaldo, J. R., Sharrow, S. O., Timonen, T. and Herberman, R. B. (1981). *J. Immun.* In press.

Perussia, B. and Trinchieri, G. (1981). *J. Immun.* **126**, 754.

Perussia, B., Mangoni, L., Engers, H. D. and Trinchieri, G. (1980). *J. Immun.* **125**, 1589.

Reid, L. M., Minato, N., Gresser, I., Holland, J., Kadish, A. and Bloom, B. R. (1981). *Proc. natn. Acad. Sci. U.S.A.* **78**, 1171.

Roder, J. C. and Duwe, A. (1979). *Nature, Lond.* **278**, 451.

Roder, J. C. and Haliotis, T. (1981). *Immunology Today* **96**.

Roder, J. C., Kiessling, P., Biberfeld, P. and Andersson, B. (1978). *J. Immun.* **121**, 2509.

Roder, J. C., Laing, L., Haliotis, T. and Kozbor, D. (1981). *In* "NK cells: Fundamental Aspects and Role in Cancer" (Eds R. B. Herberman, C. Rosenfeld and B. Serrou). Human Cancer Immunology, Vol. 6. North-Holland, Amsterdam.

Saksela, E. and Timonen, T. (1980). *In* "Natural Cell-mediated Immunity Against Tumors" (Ed. R. B. Herberman) p. 173. Academic Press, New York.

Saksela, E., Timonen, T. and Cantell, K. (1979a). *Scand. J. Immun.* **10**, 257.

Saksela, E., Timonen, T., Ranki, A-M. and Häyry, P. (1979b). *Immun. Rev.* **44**, 71.

Saksela, E., Timonen, T. and Cantell, K. (1980). *Ann. N.Y. Acad. Sci.* **350**, 102.

Saksela, E., Tarkkanen, J., Carpén, O. and Virtanen, I. (1981).

Santoni, A., Riccardi, C., Barlozzari, T. and Herberman, R. B. (1980). *Int. J. Cancer* **26**, 837.

Savary, C. A. and Lotzova, E. (1978). *J. Immun.* **120**, 239.

Seeley, J. K. and Golub, S. H. (1978). *J. Immun.* **120**, 1415.

Silva, A., Bonavida, B. and Targan, S. (1980). *J. Immun.* **125**, 479.

Stutman, O. (1980). *In* "Natural Cell-mediated Immunity Against Tumors" (Ed. R. B. Herberman) p. 231. Academic Press, New York.

Stutman, O. and Cuttito, M. J. (1981). *Nature, Lond.* **290**, 254.

Takasugi, M., Mickey, M. R. and Terasaki, P. I. (1973). *Cancer Res.* **33**, 2898.

Talmadge, J. E., Meyers, K. M., Prieur, D. J. and Starkey, J. R. (1980). *Nature, Lond.* **284**, 622.

Targan, S. and Dorey, F. (1980). *J. Immun.* **124**, 2157.

Tarkkanen, J. and Saksela, E. (1981). *Scand. J. Immun.* In press.

Tarkkanen, J., Timonen, T. and Saksela, E. (1980). *Scand. J. Immun.* **11**, 383.

Tarkkanen, J., Saksela, E. and Cantell, K. (1981). In preparation.

Timonen, T., Saksela, E., Ranki, A-M. and Häyry, P. (1979). *Cell. Immun.* **48**, 133.

Timonen, T., Saksela, E., Virtanen, I. and Cantell, K. (1980). *Eur. J. Immun.* **10**, 422.

Timonen, T., Ortaldo, J. R. and Herberman, R. B. (1981a). *J. exp. Med.* In press.

Timonen, T., Ortaldo, J. R. and Herberman, R. B. (1981b). In preparation.

Tötterman, T., Häyry, P., Saksela, E., Timonen, T. and Eklund, B. (1978). *Eur. J. Immun.* **8**, 872.

Trinchieri, G., Santoli, D., Dee, R. R. and Knowles, B. (1978). *J. exp. Med.* **147**, 1299.

Trinchieri, G. and Santoli, D. (1978). *J. exp. Med.* **147**, 1314.

Tursz, T. (1981). *In* "NK cells: Fundamental Aspects and Role in Cancer" (Eds Cl. Rosenfeld, R. B. Herberman and B. Serrou). Human Cancer Immunology, Vol. 6. North-Holland, Amsterdam.

Vanky, F., Argov, S. and Klein, E. (1981). *Int. J. Cancer* **27**, 273.

Virelizier, J. L., Lipinski, M., Tursz, T. and Criscelli, C. (1979). *Lancet* **ii**, 696.

Welsh, R. M. (1978). *J. exp. Med.* **148**, 163.

Welsh, R. M., Kärre, K., Hansson, M., Kunkel, L. A. and Kiessling, R. W. (1981). *J. Immun.* **126**, 219.

Genetic Control of the Interferon System

DORIS L. SLATE AND FRANK H. RUDDLE

Department of Biology, Yale University, New Haven, Connecticut, USA and *Central Research, Pfizer Incorporated, Groton, Connecticut, USA*

Y. H. TAN

Department of Medical Biochemistry, University of Calgary, Calgary, Alberta, Canada

I INTRODUCTION

Somatic cell genetic techniques have proven to be valuable in the elucidation of the genetic regulation of interferon production and response. Studies using interspecific cell hybrids and cell variants have provided information regarding chromosomal assignments for genes involved in the human and mouse interferon systems (Slate and Ruddle, 1979a).

Recent advances in the molecular biology of the interferon system, the purification of interferons, the use of pure interferon as immunogen, and the cloning of interferon genes, will provide new tools for the genetic analysis of interferon synthesis and its response. It is now clear that the interferon systems involve multigene families; not only are there antigenically distinct classes of interferon molecules (for example, the human α, β, and γ classes), but within a given class there are multiple protein species encoded by separate genes.

We wish to review the contributions made by somatic cell genetic analysis to the understanding of interferon as a multifamily gene system, and to suggest some possible directions for future work.

II GENETIC CONTROL OF INTERFERON SENSITIVITY

A Somatic Cell Genetic Studies

Since interferon synthesis and action are inducible phenotypes which can be studied in tissue culture cells, somatic cell genetic techniques can be employed to define and map loci involved in the interferon system. Limited species specificity (human interferons generally being more active on human cells than on mouse cells and vice versa) suggested the use of human/mouse somatic cell hybrids for mapping purposes.

Experiments with human/mouse cell hybrids segregating human chromosomes indicated a concordant segregation of the interferon induced "antiviral protein" and "indophenol oxidase B" (cytoplasmic superoxide dismutase). These genes were assigned to human chromosome 21 (Tan *et al.*, 1973; Chany *et al.*, 1975). Tan *et al.* (1974b) then examined the effect of chromosome 21 dosage on the expression of the human interferon-induced antiviral state. The amount of interferon required to induce the antiviral state in human diploid cell lines was 3–7 times higher than that which was effective on trisomy 21 cell lines; monosomy 21 cells required even more interferon (Tan, 1975).

Although the usual pattern for chromosome segregation in human/rodent cell hybrids involves the preferential loss of human chromosomes, "reverse" segregant hybrids can be constructed by fusing primary mouse cells to transformed human cells. Using this approach, Lin *et al.* (1980) mapped the mouse gene responsible for conferring sensitivity to interferon to murine chromosome 16. Cox *et al.* (1980) have also mapped the mouse interferon sensitivity gene to chromosome 16 using mouse/Chinese hamster hybrids segregating mouse chromosomes. Both groups found a syntenic relationship for the genes coding for mouse interferon sensitivity and cytoplasmic superoxide dismutase as was previously reported for the corresponding human genes.

B Possible Role of Interferon Receptors

The product(s) of the gene(s) on human chromosome 21 (and the corresponding gene on mouse chromosome 16) responsible for conferring interferon sensitivity has not been isolated, although Wiranowska-Stewart and Stewart (1977) have suggested a cell surface receptor for interferon because different levels of interferon binding could be recorded for cells with different numbers of copies of human chromosome 21. However such measurements did not differentiate between the specific and nonspecific binding of interferon to cells. Binding studies using labelled purified interferons (see Aguet, 1980; Branca and Baglioni, in press) are now revealing the characteristics of interferon receptors.

Slate *et al.* (1978) demonstrated that a human/mouse somatic cell hybrid retaining human chromosome 21 as the only detectable human genetic material could respond to human leukocyte and fibroblast interferons. The response was measured by antiviral activity assays and by assessing biochemical changes in extracts from interferon treated cells. Human interferon treatment could trigger mouse specific changes in this hybrid cell line.

Injecting mice with human/mouse somatic cell hybrids results in the production of antibodies which are directed against human cell surface components, provided that the mice are of the same strain as the murine parent of the hybrid. Antibodies raised against hybrid cells containing human chromosomes 4, 21 and 22 could block the action of human interferon on diploid human fibroblasts (Revel *et al.*, 1976). This blocking activity was more pronounced in monosomy 21 cells and decreased as the number of copies of chromosome 21 increased in the target cell. Pre-adsorption of the antibody on cells with chromosome 21 could remove its blocking activity, while pre-absorption on cells retaining chromosomes 4 and 22 (but lacking 21) could not. These studies have been extended to antisera raised against human/mouse hybrid cells retaining human chromosomes 21 and 22 or 21 alone with similar results (Slate and Ruddle, 1978).

Recently monoclonal antibodies, directed against chromosome 21-coded cell surface antigens, which block the action of human interferon, have been produced (Kamarck *et al.*, 1981) by the method of Kohler and Milstein (1975). Spleen cells from mice injected with a human/mouse hybrid line retaining only human chromosome 21 were fused with established mouse myeloma cells, and three hybridomas with interferon blocking activity were isolated (Slate *et al.*, in preparation). The antibodies must be incubated with human cells before the addition of human interferon in order to exhibit blocking activity. The activity of both leukocyte (α) and fibroblast (β) interferon can be blocked by the antibodies, while that of immune (γ) interferon cannot.

These results suggest that human interferon sensitivity is determined by a gene on chromosome 21 coding for a cell surface receptor for human interferon. With the availability of purified, radioactively labelled human interferons it is now possible to demonstrate the existence of specific cell surface receptors for human interferon (Branca and Baglioni, in press); this has recently been done by Aguet (1980) for the mouse interferon receptor. The monoclonal antibodies which block interferon action should prove useful in isolating and characterizing the putative human interferon receptor(s).

The structure of the postulated human interferon receptor(s) has been the subject of several studies (see Chany, 1976; Kohn, 1978). Ganglioside and glycoprotein components have been suggested for the receptor, with a membrane re-arrangement being required to transmit the signal of interferon binding at the membrane to the cell nucleus to initiate the cellular alterations known as the antiviral state. The binding of several agents such a cholera toxin and thyrotropic hormone can block the antiviral activity of interferon, presumably by blocking accessibility of interferon receptors. Kohn *et al.* (1976) has suggested that these results predict a similarity in the receptors for these agents and interferon.

Studies with mutant cells which no longer respond to one type of human or mouse interferon (see, for example, Bourgeade *et al.*, 1980; Ankel *et al.*, 1980) are providing clues about the activities of different species of interferons. If the α and β interferons share a common receptor the sequences of purified α and β interferons should reveal the regions of the molecule responsible for receptor binding. In fact, homologies at the nucleotide and amino acid sequence levels have been described for human α and β interferons (Taniguchi *et al.*, 1980). Hybrid interferon molecules made with the amino terminus of one interferon subtype and the carboxy terminus of another (R. Lawn, ICN-UCLA Symposia, Developmental Biology Using Purified Genes, 1981; Streuli *et al.*, 1981) may provide details about the molecular structure of the interferon molecule and define the basis for species specificity and cross-species activity. In these studies, the molecular biology and biochemistry of interferon gene cloning and purification complement the findings made with somatic cell hybrids and mutants.

III INTERFERONS COMPRISE A MULTIGENE FAMILY

A Somatic Cell Genetic Studies

Within a given animal species several antigenically distinct types of interferon can be produced, depending on the cell type and inducing stimulus. In the human interferon system three major antigenic types of interferon have been described: α (leukocyte), β (fibroblast) and γ (immune). α interferons are usually produced by buffy coat leukocytes or established lymphoblastoid cells following virus induction. β Interferon is usually made in cultured fibroblasts after induction with double stranded RNA. γ Interferon is usually produced by T cells after mitogenic or antigenic stimulation. A single cell type may produce more than one type of interferon: for example, human fibroblasts produce a mixture of α and β interferons after virus induction (Havell *et al.*, 1978), and mouse Ehrlich ascites tumour cells produce two β-like and one α-like interferons after Newcastle disease virus infection (Taira *et al.*, 1980).

Somatic cell genetic studies thus far have produced several chromosomal assignments for human interferon genes. Tan *et al.* (1974a) found that human chromosomes 2 and 5 were necessary for human interferon production in human/mouse somatic cell hybrids. More recent studies have suggested that chromosome 5 alone (Morgan and Faik, 1977; Tan *et al.*, 1977) is responsible for human interferon production. Slate and Ruddle (1979b) found evidence for separate fibroblast interferon loci on chromosomes 2 and 5. Meager *et al.* (1979a, b) have presented data for a single fibroblast interferon locus on human chromosome 9.

B Information from Gene Cloning

There are two questions which are immediately evident from the above discussion: Why have all the assignments been for fibroblast interferon loci, and why do the assignments disagree? The explanation most often given for the mapping of only fibroblast interferon loci is that the nonsegregating mouse parent used in generating the human/mouse hybrids is usually a fibroblast line and tends to "dominate" the interferon phenotype (Burke, 1980). Human/mouse hybrid cells produce human fibroblast interferon even when the human parent is a peripheral blood leukocyte, which reflects the rescue of genetic expression as a result of somatic cell hybridization. Perhaps the use of differentiated lymphoid cell lines as nonsegregating parents in human/rodent hybrids will allow expression of other interferon genes; on the other hand, since the recent cloning of human interferon cDNAs and genomic sequences, mapping these genes is no longer dependent on having human interferon genes expressed in a hybrid cell.

DNA from a panel of human/rodent hybrid cells, each well characterized for human chromosome content, is isolated and digested with several restriction endonucleases. The digests are electrophoresed on agarose gels to fractionate the DNA fragments on the basis of size, and the DNA is then transferred to filters by Southern blotting (Southern, 1975). A radioactive interferon sequence probe is then hybridized to the DNA on the filters. Human and rodent specific hybridization patterns are identified, and the hybrid cells analysed for their hybridization patterns, either rodent alone or a composite of rodent and human patterns. By correlating the presence of given human chromosomes with the appearance of human specific restriction fragments, genes for interferon can be mapped to specific chromosomes. Using this approach, a family of α interferon sequences and one β interferon gene have been mapped to human chromosome 9 (Owerbach *et al.*, 1981; Slate *et al.*, submitted for publication; Pitha *et al.*, submitted for publication). Progress in this area of gene mapping which combines recombinant DNA technology and somatic cell genetics is rapid, and information concerning multiple chromosomal assignments is given below.

C Multiple Interferon mRNAs and Proteins

As discussed above, interferons comprise a multigene family (see Goeddel *et al.*, 1981; Weissenbach *et al.*, 1980). Furthermore the heterogeneity of interferon genes is reflected in the synthesis of multiple interferon mRNAs for β interferon (Sehgal and Sagar, 1980; Soreq *et al.*, 1981; Sehgal, 1981) and α interferon (Sagar *et al.*, 1981; Sehgal *et al.*, 1981a, b) and multiple α (Rubinstein *et al.*, 1979) and β (Inoue *et al.*, 1981; Nyari *et al.*, 1981) interferon proteins. The earlier gene assignments for interferon to chromosomes 2, 5 and 9 probably reflect this multiplicity of interferon genes. Several human β interferon mRNA species have been found in induced human/mouse somatic cell hybrids. Tentative gene assignments for these mRNAs have been made (β_1 to chromosome 9, β_2 to chromosome 5, β_3 and β_5 to chromosome 2), but the regulation of these mRNAs is complex (Sagar, Slate, Ruddle, and Sehgal, manuscript in preparation), and is still under active investigation.

Further studies with somatic cell hybrids should reveal the chromosomal location of each of the genes responsible for the production of a given interferon mRNA and protein species. The organization of interferon genes in the genome poses an interesting biological regulation problem. A set of the human α interferon genes and at least one β interferon gene appear to lack introns and map to chromosome 9. The β_2 interferon gene (Weissenbach *et al.*, 1980) may have introns, codes for an mRNA which does not cross-hybridize with β_1 mRNA, and maps to a different chromosome. There may also be other human interferon gene clusters yet undiscovered.

IV REGULATION OF INTERFERON SYNTHESIS

A Type of Interferon made in Cell Hybrids

Somatic cell hybrids have proven useful in studying the regulation of differentiated cell functions (see, for example, Brown and Weiss, 1975). Extinction or activation of certain differentiated traits can be observed in hybrids between two differentiated cell types or between a differentiated cell and an "undifferentiated" transformed fibroblast line.

As discussed above, the human/rodent somatic cell hybrids examined to date have produced human fibroblast interferon, and not leukocyte or immune interferon. The rodent parental lines used in mapping studies have been mouse or Chinese hamster fibroblasts, and their phenotype may influence the type of interferon made in hybrids. The response of hybrid cells to different inducers has also been examined (see Slate and Ruddle, 1979b; Burke, 1980); the role of the rodent parent here is not clear.

Construction of human/rodent hybrids where both parents are of lymphoid origin may permit the study of human α and γ gene expression. Isolating and maintaining such hybrids will be more difficult than culturing fibroblast hybrids, however.

B Superinduction

Many investigators have described protocols for interferon induction employing poly (rI) · poly (rC) and suitably timed doses of metabolic inhibitors which block transcription and translation (see Tan *et al.*, 1970; Vilček and Ng, 1971; Sehgal *et al.*, 1976). These protocols result in "superinduction" of interferon: the amounts of interferon mRNA and protein produced are increased. It has been reported that chromosome 16 plays a role in superinduction of interferon synthesis (Creagan *et al.*, 1975). This assignment should be confirmed, and the effects of the superinduction protocol should be tested for α and γ interferon synthesis as well.

Somatic cell hybrids may prove useful in identifying factors which control the half-life of interferon mRNA and the translatability of interferon mRNA. There are several factors which have been suggested in the regulation of interferon synthesis, vis. a post-transcriptional regulation (Tan *et al.*, 1970) or a transcriptional regulation (Tan and Berthold, 1977; Marcus, 1981).

C Gene Transfer

Recent advances in DNA-mediated gene transfer in mammalian cells allow the introduction of small amounts of genetic material into somatic cells in culture. Weissmann (ICN-UCLA Symposia, Developmental Biology Using Purified Genes, 1981) has reported that introduction of cloned human α interferon DNA into mouse cells results initially in transient expression of the human interferon genes. After integration of the DNA into the recipient genome, the introduced interferon genes are again under inducible regulation with virus induction required for their expression. This exciting development suggests that the expression of interferon genes can be studied in different cell backgrounds to examine the effect of different recipient cell phenotypes on the expression of α, β and γ genes, for example.

Direct micro-injection (see Diacumakos, 1973; Liu *et al.*, 1979) or other modes of uptake of nucleic acids into somatic cells can also be used to study transcription or translation of interferon DNA or mRNA. While constitutive interferon production may be deleterious to cells because of interferon's known growth inhibitory effects, genetic engineering of the appropriate regulatory sequence on cellular DNA may result in higher or constitutive interferon production by cells.

V TRANSFER OF ANTIVIRAL STATE BETWEEN CELLS

Blalock and Baron (1977) have reported that if cells of two different animal species, whose interferons exhibit species specificity, are co-cultivated after treatment with one parental interferon, the antiviral state can be observed in both cell types. They postulated that there can be a transfer of the antiviral state between the cells.

The most likely means of transfer, given the requirement for intimate association of the co-cultivated cells, would be via the junctions. One possible way to test this hypothesis is outlined below. Some mouse L cells have a defect in the formation functional gap junctions; this defect can be corrected by a human gene when the defective mouse cells are fused to normal human fibroblasts to form hybrid cells. If a small molecule, such as the endoribonuclease activator pppA2′p5′A2′p5′A (Kerr *et al.*, 1977), is transferred between cells to produce an antiviral state, co-cultivation of such a hybrid (gap junction forming, but lacking human chromosome 21 so that it cannot respond to human interferon) with human fibroblasts could be used to study the transfer. Treating the mixed culture with human or mouse interferon should protect both cell types, while treating co-cultivated mouse L cells and human fibroblasts with either type of interferon should only protect one cell type.

VI INTERFERON, HORMONES AND ENDORPHINS

A Possible Structural Relatedness

Several intriguing reports have suggested that interferon can mimic the effects of certain hormones and vice versa (see, for example, Blalock and Stanton, 1980). Blalock and Smith (1980) have suggested that interferons contain sequences related to, or identical with, ACTH and endorphins. ACTH and endorphins are normally produced in the form of a large precursor polypeptide, pro-opiomelanocortin, which is cleaved to give various hormones and neuropeptides (Chang *et al.*, 1980). Since both the pro-opiomelanocortin and several interferon genes have been sequenced, it should be possible to determine if there is a structural relatedness between interferon and these small peptides. Wc (Slate and Ruddle) have stated such an analysis, working on the following assumptions: the ACTH and endorphin sequences should bear the same positional relationship in any interferon precursor as in the normal pro-opiomelanocortin sequence, and ACTH, which can be cleaved from Blalock's precursor, should be at one end of the α interferon sequence. The results of our analysis thus far are suggestive, but not definitive, of some homology.

B Mechanism of Action

As discussed earlier, certain hormones and toxins can block the binding of interferon to cells and the development of the antiviral state (Kohn, 1978). It has been suggested that this may reflect a similarity in the receptor structures for interferon and these agents. Given the findings that hormones may induce an antiviral state, and that interferon may elicit responses normally induced by hormones, it may be that the signals transmitted to the nucleus after membrane binding of these agents may be similar if not identical. Somatic cells which have mutant responses to interferon or one of these agents can be studied to determine if the defect is at the level of signal reception or transmission of the signal to alter cellular physiology. Making hybrids between such mutants and normal cells will allow the dissection of the genetics behind these processes.

VII PROSPECTS

By combining techniques from somatic cell genetics and recombinant DNA technology, we should see a tremendous increase in our knowledge of the interferon system in the near future. The development of cell mutants in interferon production and response, and the complementation of these mutations by somatic cell hybridization, should reveal new aspects of the genetic regulation of these processes. A comparison of hormone and interferon gene and protein sequences should allow us to determine if there is a structural basis for their similarity of action in some systems. The study of hybrid interferon molecules should tell us much about the molecular basis of interferon binding and species specificity. Gene transfer experiments should allow us to modify interferon genetic regulation and monitor for altered expression in recipient cells. The next few years will be very exciting ones in the use of the interferon system as a model to study mammalian genetic regulations.

VIII ACKNOWLEDGEMENTS

We wish to thank Drs M. Kamarck and P. D'Eustachio for discussions about monoclonal antibodies and mapping interferon genes using recombinant DNA approaches, and Dr T. K. Wong for discussions about gene transfer and genetic regulation. DLS was supported by a Leukemia Society of America Postdoctoral Fellowship. YHT has been supported by the Canadian Medical Research Council and USPHS grant CA-19721. Interferon research in the lab of FHR has been supported by NIH grant GM09966 and American Cancer Society Grant CD-2. We wish to thank C. P. Chiu for typing the manuscript. Thanks also to the Fraternal Order of Eagles, Calgary for a travel grant to the authors for the writing of this manuscript.

IX REFERENCES

Aguet, M. (1980). *Nature, Lond.* **284**, 459–461.

Ankel, H., Krishnamurti, C., Besancon, F., Stefanos, S. and Falcoff, E. (1980). *Proc. natn. Acad. Sci. U.S.A.* **77**, 2528–2532.

Blalock, J. E. and Baron, S. (1977). *Nature, Lond.* **269**, 422–425.

Blalock, J. E. and Smith, E. M. (1980). *Proc. natn. Acad. Sci. U.S.A.* **77**, 5972–5974.

Blalock, J. E. and Stanton, J. D. (1980). *Nature, Lond.* **283**, 406–408.

Bourgeade, M. F., Chany, C. and Merigan, T. C. (1980). *J. gen. Virol.* **46**, 449–454.

Brown, J. E. and Weiss, M. C. (1975). *Cell* **6**, 481–494.

Burke, D. C. (1980). *In* "Interferon 1980" (Ed. I. Gresser) Vol. 2, pp 47–64.

Chang, A. C. Y., Cochet, M. and Cohen, S. N. (1980). *Proc. natn. Acad. Sci. U.S.A.* **77**, 4890–4894.

Chany, C. (1976). *Biomed. Express* **24**, 148–157.

Chany, C., Vignal, M., Couillin, P., Cong, N. V., Boue, J. and Boue, A., (1975). *Proc. natn. Acad. Sci. U.S.A.* **72**, 3129–3133.

Cox, D. R., Epstein, L. B. and Epstein, C. J. (1980). *Proc. natn. Acad. Sci. U.S.A.* **77**, 2168–2172.

Creagan, R. P., Tan, Y. H., Chen, S. and Ruddle, F. H. (1975). *Fedn Proc. Fedn Am. Socs exp. Biol.* **34**, 2222–2226.

Diacumakos, E. G. (1973). *In* "Methods in Cell Biology" (Ed. D. M. Prescott) pp. 287–311. Academic Press, New York.

Goeddel, D. V., Leung, D. W., Dull, J. J., Gross, M., Lawn, R. M., McCandliss, R., Seeburg, P. H., Ullrich, A., Yelverton, E. and Gray, P. W. (1981). *Nature, Lond.* **290**, 20–26.

Havell, E. A., Hayes, T. G. and Vilček, J. (1978). *Virology* **89**, 330–334.

Inoue, M., Erlich, H., Nyari, L., Colby, B. and Tan, Y. H. (1981). *Antiviral Res.* **1**, 56.

Kamarck, M. E., Slate, D. L., D'Eustachio, P., Barel, B. and Ruddle, F. H. (1981). *Fedn Proc. Fedn Am. Socs exp. Biol.* **40**, 1051.

Kerr, I. M., Brown, R. E. and Hovanessian, A. G. (1977). *Nature, Lond.* **268**, 540–542.

Kohler, G. and Milstein, C. (1975). *Nature, Lond.* **256**, 495–497.

Kohn, L. D. (1978). *In* "Receptors and Recognition" (Eds P. Cuatrecasas and M. F. Greaves) Series A, Vol. 5, pp. 133–212. Chapman and Hall, London.

Kohn, L. D., Friedman, R. M., Holmes, J. M. and Lee, G. (1976). *Proc. Natn. Acad. Sci. U.S.A.* **73**, 3695–3699.

Lin, P-F., Slate, D. L., Lawyer, F. C. and Ruddle, F. H. (1980). *Science, N.Y.* **209**, 285–287.

Liu, C-P, Slate, D. L., Gravel, R. and Ruddle, F. H. (1979). *Proc. natn. Acad. Sci. U.S.A.* **76**, 4503–4506.

Marcus, P. (1981). *Tex. Rep. Biol. Med.*, in press.

Meager, A., Graves, H., Burke, D. C. and Swallow, D. M. (1979a). *Nature, Lond.* **280**, 493–495.

Meager, A., Graves, H. E., Walker, J. R., Burke, D. C., Swallow, D. M. and Westerwald, A. (1979b). *J. gen. Virol.* **45**, 309–321.

Morgan, M. J. and Faik, P. (1977). *Br. J. Cancer* **36**, 254.

Owerbach, D., Rutter, W. J., Shows, T. B., Gray, P., Goeddel, D. V. and Lawn, R. M. (1981). *Proc. natn. Acad. Sci. U.S.A.* **78**, 3123–3127.

Nyari, L., Tan, Y. H., Erlich, H. A. (1981). *Antiviral Res.* **1**, 6.

Revel, M., Bash, D. and Ruddle, F. H. (1976). *Nature, Lond.* **260**, 139–141.

Rubinstein, M., Rubinstein, S., Familletti, P. C., Miller, R. S., Waldman, A. A. and Pestka, S. (1979). *Proc. natn. Acad. Sci. U.S.A.* **76**, 640–644.

Sagar, A. D., Pickering, L. A., Sussman-Berger, P., Stewart II, W. E., and Sehgal, P. B. (1981). *Nucl. Acids Res.* **9**, 149–160.

Sehgal, P. B. (1981). *Antiviral Res.* **1**, 4.

Sehgal, P. B. and Sagar, A. D. (1980). *Nature, Lond.* **288**, 95–97.

Sehgal, P. B., Tamm, I. and Vilček, J. (1976). *Virology* **70**, 256–259.

Sehgal, P. B., Sagar, A. D., Braude, I. A. and Smith, D. (1981a). *In* "The Biology of the Interferon System" (Eds E. De Maeyer, G. Galasso and H. Schellekens) pp. 43–46. Elsevier/North-Holland, Amsterdam.

Sehgal, P. B., Sagar, A. D. and Braude, I. A. (1981b). *Science, N.Y.*, in press.

Slate, D. L. and Ruddle, F. H. (1978). *Cytogenet. Cell Genet.* **22**, 265–269.

Slate, D. L. and Ruddle, F. H. (1979a). *Pharmacol. Ther.* **4**, 221–230.

Slate, D. L. and Ruddle, F. H. (1979b). *Cell* **16**, 171–180.

Slate, D. L., Shulman, L., Lawrence, J. B., Revel, M. and Ruddle, F. H. (1978). *J. gen. Virol.* **25**, 319–325.

Soreq, H., Sagar, A. D. and Sehgal, P. B. (1981). *Proc. natn. Acad. Sci. U.S.A.* **78**, 1741–1745.

Southern, E. M. (1975). *J. molec. Biol.* **98**, 503–517.

Streuli, M., Hall, A., Boll, W., Stewart II, W. E., Nagasta, S. and Weissmann, C. (1981). *Proc. natn. Acad. Sci. U.S.A.* **78**, 2848–2852.

Taira, H., Broeze, R. J., Jayaram, B. M., Lengyel, P., Hunkapiller, M. W. and Hood, L. E. (1980). *Science, N.Y.* **207**, 528–530.

Tan, Y. H. (1975). *Nature, Lond.* **253**, 280–282.

Tan, Y. H. and Berthold, W. (1977). *J. gen. Virol.* **34**, 401–412.

Tan, Y. H., Armstrong, J. A., Ke, Y. H. and Ho, M. (1970). *Proc. natn. Acad. Sci. U.S.A.* **67**, 464–471.

Tan, Y. H., Tischfield, J. A. and Ruddle, F. H. (1973). *J. exp. Med.* **137**, 317–330.
Tan, Y. H., Creagan, R. P. and Ruddle, F. H. (1974a). *Proc. natn. Acad. Sci. U.S.A.* **71**, 2251–2255.
Tan, Y. H., Schneider, E. L., Tischfield, J., Epstein, C. J. and Ruddle, F. H. (1974b). *Science, N.Y.* **186**, 61–63.
Tan, Y. H., Tan, C. and Berthold, W. (1977). *Tex. Rep. Biol. Med.* **35**, 63–68.
Taniguchi, T., Mantei, N., Schwartzstein, M., Nagata, S., Muramatsu, M. and Weissmann, C. (1980). *Nature, Lond.* **285**, 547–549.
Vilček, J. and Ng, M. H. (1971). *J. gen. Virol.* **7**, 588–594.
Weissenbach, J., Chernajovsky, Y., Zeevi, M., Shulman, L., Soreq, H., Nir, U., Wallach, D., Perricaudet, M., Tiollais, P. and Revel, M. (1980). *Proc. natn. Acad. Sci. U.S.A.* **77**, 7152–7156.
Wiranowska-Stewart, M. and Stewart II, W. E. (1977). *J. gen. Virol.* **37**, 629–633.

Mechanisms of Interferon Action: The (2′–5′)(A)$_n$ Synthetase–RNase L Pathway

PETER LENGYEL

Department of Molecular Biophysics and Biochemistry, Yale University, New Haven, Connecticut, USA

I INTRODUCTION

The various activities of interferons (e.g. antiviral, cell growth regulatory and immunomodulatory) appear to be mediated by several biochemical mechanisms (Stewart, 1979; Taylor-Papadimitriou, 1980; Vilček *et al.*, 1980). Among those that have been proposed so far, e.g. acceleration of RNA cleavage (Brown *et al.*, 1976), alteration of mRNA methylation (Sen *et al.*, 1975; Kahana *et al.*, 1981), inhibition of peptide chain initiation (Lebleu *et al.*, 1976; Roberts *et al.*, 1976; Zilberstein *et al.*, 1976; Farrell *et al.*, 1978), and protein glycosylation (Maheshwari *et al.*, 1980), the best characterized is the pathway resulting in an accelerated RNA cleavage. Here we will survey our present understanding of this pathway (Fig. 1) together with some of the findings, often serendipitous which have contributed to this.

II INHIBITION OF REOVIRUS REPLICATION BY INTERFERONS

Many of the experiments on the biochemistry of interferon action in the early 1970s aimed to discover the mechanism(s) by which the replication of viruses is impaired by interferons. The questions usually asked were which steps in the replication of a particular virus in a particular cell were blocked or which were the viral components or virus-specific molecules whose accumulation was diminished in cells treated with interferons.

During this period most of the work of my colleagues and me at Yale concerning this problem has been done with mouse (L929 or Ehrlich ascites tumour) cells and reovirus (Graziadei *et al.*, 1973; Gupta *et al.*, 1974). This virus has a double stranded RNA genome consisting of 10 different segments (Joklik, 1974). After penetration into the cell the virions are converted into "subviral" particles by the removal and cleavage of some of their outer coat proteins. This results in the activation of various virion-associated enzymes. The activated enzymes in the subviral particles synthesize and release 10 types of reo mRNAs into the cytoplasm. In this the mRNAs are translated into viral proteins. These assemble into particles, everyone of which contains one of each of the 10 species of reo mRNAs. Within each particle 10 genomic double stranded RNAs are formed by the

$$\text{(1)}\quad (n+1)\,\text{ATP} \xrightarrow[\text{double stranded RNA}]{(2'\text{-}5')(\text{A})_n\ \text{synthetase}} (2'\text{-}5')(\text{A})_{n+1}{}^{*} + n\ \text{pyrophosphate}$$

$$\text{(2)}\quad \text{RNase L}^{\ddagger}\ (\text{latent}) \underset{-(2'\text{-}5')(\text{A})_n}{\overset{+(2'\text{-}5')(\text{A})_n}{\rightleftharpoons}} \text{RNase L (activated)}$$

Fig. 1. The $(2'\text{-}5')(\text{A})_n$ synthetase-RNase L pathway.

* $(2'\text{-}5')(\text{A})_n$ have 5′ terminal triphosphates thus a more revealing formula for these compounds is $(2'\text{-}5')\text{pppA}(\text{pA})_n$. n varies from 1 to about 15.

‡The same enzyme is also sometimes designated as RNase F.

synthesis of one complementary RNA strand along each of the 10 viral mRNAs. The resulting particles (provirions) can either synthesize further reo mRNAs and thereby amplify the yield of virus replication or can complete their outer coat by binding further capsid proteins and thereby mature into infectious virions (Joklik, 1974).

We established that the treatment of L929 cells with interferons does not affect the early steps of reovirus replication, i.e. the adsorption to cells, penetration into cells and partial uncoating of the virions to form subviral particles. It did impair, however, the accumulation of reovirus specific mRNAs, double stranded RNAs and proteins (Galster and Lengyel, 1976; see also Wiebe and Joklik, 1975). A reduction of viral RNA accumulation in interferon-treated cells infected with SV40, vesicular stomatitis virus, vaccinia virus or frog polyhedral cytoplasmic deoxyribovirus had been reported even earlier (Marcus *et al.*, 1971; Oxman and Levine, 1971; Bialy and Colby, 1972; Gravell and Cromeans, 1972; Manders *et al.*, 1972).

III ACCELERATED DEGRADATION OF RNA IN EXTRACTS FROM INTERFERON-TREATED CELLS: DEPENDENCE ON DOUBLE STRANDED RNA AND ATP

The impairment of reovirus RNA accumulation in interferon-treated cells prompted us to compare the rate of reo mRNA degradation in extracts from cells treated with interferon to that in extracts from control cells. For this purpose reo mRNAs were generated *in vitro* by incubating activated reovirus (i.e. reovirions treated with chymotrypsin to activate the virion-associated RNA synthesizing enzymes) with ribonucleoside triphosphates. The reo mRNA preparation isolated from this incubation was slightly contaminated with reovirus genomic double stranded RNA. The reo mRNAs in this preparation were degraded faster when incubated in an extract from interferon-treated cells than when incubated in an extract from control cells (Brown *et al.*, 1976). Upon finding this rate difference we decided to invest the labour needed to isolate pure reo mRNAs (i.e. free of double stranded RNA) and repeat the experiments.

To our dismay the extract from interferon-treated cells and that from control cells cleaved the pure (double stranded RNA-free) mRNA preparation at the same rate. We were elated to find, however, that the re-addition of double stranded RNA to the incubation mixture restored the difference: It accelerated the cleavage in the extract from interferon-treated cells but did not affect that in the extract from control cells (Brown *et al.*, 1976). An extract from interferon-treated human (HeLa) cells responded to double stranded RNA in the same way as that from an extract from interferon-treated mouse (Ehrlich ascites tumour) cells and a synthetic double stranded RNA (poly I: poly C) had the same effect as reovirus genomic double stranded RNA (Brown *et al.*, 1976; Shaila *et al.*, 1977).

The experiments on RNA degradation had been performed in conditions of protein synthesis, i.e. in reaction mixtures supplemented with amino acids, ATP and GTP. Experiments involving the omission of these supplements, one type at a time, revealed that the acceleration of RNA cleavage in the extracts from interferon-treated cells also required ATP (Sen *et al.*, 1976). To establish whether double stranded RNA and ATP need be present when reo mRNA is cleaved or if they serve only to activate an otherwise latent nuclease (which after activation does not require the presence of these two agents any more) we performed the following tests. We incubated the extracts from interferon-treated cells first with ATP alone or double stranded RNA alone or with double stranded RNA as well as ATP. Thereafter we destroyed ATP (by converting it to ADP by treatment with hexokinase and glucose) and degraded the double stranded RNA (by incubating it with the enzyme RNase III which cleaves it into short segments which, as we demonstrated separately, do not affect RNA cleavage). Finally we added reo mRNA (and if these had not been present during the first incubation either ATP or double stranded RNA) and tested for the rate of RNA cleavage. The results indicated that (a) neither double stranded RNA nor ATP are required during the mRNA cleavage but (b) both have to be present during the first incubation. Thus these two agents are needed only for the activation of a latent nuclease (Sen *et al.*, 1976).

Having divided the functioning of the nuclease system into two steps (1, activation of a latent nuclease; 2, RNA cleavage by the activated nuclease) we proceeded to divide the cell extract into complementary components. This was accomplished by fractionation on an ion exchange column (DEAE cellulose). One of the fractions (DE1), if incubated with ATP and double stranded RNA, gave rise to a product (that we designated as ''nuclease activator'') which even after boiling the incubated reaction mixture to inactivate the enzyme(s) in fraction DE1 could activate in the second fraction (DE2) a latent nuclease (that we designated as RNase L, L standing for latent). As determined by gel filtration this ''nuclease activator'' is a low molecular weight compound (Ratner *et al.*, 1978).

The characteristics of the nuclease activator (synthesis in extracts from interferon-treated cells if supplemented with ATP and double stranded RNA, thermostability, and low molecular weight) (Ratner *et al.*, 1978) reminded us of an important finding of Kerr and his colleagues (Hovanessian *et al.*, 1977; Kerr and Brown, 1978). They discovered that (1) an extract from interferon-treated cells supplemented with double stranded RNA transforms ATP into a set of novel compounds: (2′–5′) oligoadenylates with 5′ terminal triphosphate residues; (2) these compounds are potent inhibitors of protein synthesis in cell extracts. The mechanism of action of these compounds, however, was unknown at that time. We wondered if our ''nuclease activator'' is identical with the (2′–5′) linked oligoadenylates and, if so, if it would inhibit protein synthesis by activating the latent endonuclease. We found that the answer to both of these questions was yes (Farrell *et al.*, 1978; Ratner *et al.*, 1978).

Independently Clemens and Williams (1978) reported that $(2'–5')(A)_n$ added to a rabbit reticulocyte lysate accelerates the decrease of the translatability of mRNA during incubation, and Baglioni *et al.* (1978) established that the addition of $(2'–5')(A)_n$ to an extract from HeLa cells accelerates RNA cleavage.

All these data are consistent with the existence in extracts from interferon-treated cells of the biochemical pathway shown in Fig. 1. Before proceeding to the details of this pathway we will note briefly earlier studies on the involvement of double stranded RNA in the modulation of the interferon system.

IV DOUBLE STRANDED RNA AND THE INTERFERON SYSTEM: OBSERVATIONS BEFORE 1977

In the course of searching for agents eliciting interferon production, Hilleman and his colleagues discovered in 1967 that double stranded RNA of synthetic or natural origin is a potent inducer (Field *et al.*, 1967). This finding served as a basis for a hypothesis according to which the interferon inducer in virus infected cells may be viral double stranded RNA formed in the course of virus multiplication as an intermediate (or side product) of viral RNA replication.

The ability of double stranded RNA to induce interferon production in cell culture was found to increase together with its toxicity as tested in mice

(DeClercq *et al.*, 1972). Furthermore Stewart *et al.* (1972) reported that treatment of (mouse L) cells with interferon increases their sensitivity to (i.e. makes them more prone to lysis by) double stranded RNA. In an unrelated line of research Ehrenfeld and Hunt (1971) established that virus specific double stranded RNA is the agent in the cytoplasm of poliovirus infected HeLa cells which if added to a rabbit reticulocyte lysate inhibits peptide chain initiation. Synthetic double stranded RNA has the same inhibitory action in this system as virus specific double stranded RNA.

These and other findings prompted Kerr *et al.* (1974) to compare protein synthesis in extracts from interferon-treated and control cells for sensitivity to inhibition by double stranded RNA. Their finding that protein synthesis in an extract from interferon-treated cells is more prone to inhibition by double stranded RNA than that in an extract from control cells was followed by studies revealing the formation of $(2'–5')(A)_n$ as an inhibitor of protein synthesis in extracts from interferon-treated cells supplemented with double stranded RNA.

V THE $(2'–5')(A)_n$ SYNTHETASE–RNase L PATHWAY: ENZYMES

A $(2'–5')(A)_n$ Synthetase

We isolated pure enzyme catalysing $(2'–5')(A)_n$ synthesis (reaction 1 in Fig. 1) at first from mouse Ehrlich ascites tumour cells and then from human HeLa cells (Dougherty *et al.*, 1980; Yang *et al.*, 1981). Partially purified $(2'–5')(A)_n$ synthetases were isolated from mouse L929 cells, chicken cells and rabbit reticulocytes (Ball and White, 1979; Hovanessian and Kerr, 1979; Justesen *et al.*, 1980a).

The mouse enzyme was purified 2600-fold from an extract of interferon-treated mouse Ehrlich ascites tumour cells by differential salt precipitation and ion exchange chromatography (Dougherty *et al.*, 1980). The molecular weight of the homogeneous enzyme is 105 000 as determined by gel electrophoresis in the presence of sodium dodecyl sulphate and 85 000 as determined by sedimentation through a glycerol gradient. These data indicate that (at least prior to activation by double stranded RNA) the enzyme exists as a monomer. In the presence of double stranded RNA the purified enzyme can convert the large majority (over 97%) of the ATP added to $(2'–5')(A)_n$ (where n extends from 1 to about 15) and pyrophosphate. The stoichiometry of the reaction can be shown to be

$$(n + 1)\,\text{ATP} \text{ —— } (2'–5')\text{pppA}(\text{pA})_n + n\,\text{pyrophosphate}$$

($(2'–5')$pppA$(pA)_n$ stands for the same series of compounds that are abbreviated otherwise as $(2'–5')(A)_n$. The different abbreviation is used here to emphasize that the terminus of $(2'-5')(A)_n$ is a triphosphate (Samanta *et al.*, 1980).)

It is notable (and was unexpected) that the equilibrium of the reaction is strongly shifted in favour of synthesis since the reaction does not require "pulling" by cleavage of pyrophosphate. This seems to indicate that the free energy of (2′–5′) linked oligoadenylates is different from that of (3′–5′) linked oligoadenylates (Samanta *et al.*, 1980). It may be in line with this conclusion that, as revealed by nuclear magnetic resonance and circular dichroism studies, (2′–5′) linked oligoadenylates have a stronger tendency to stack than the corresponding 3′–5′ compounds (Doornbos *et al.*, 1981).

Among the products of the enzyme, di-, tri- and tetraadenylates are usually the most abundant. The amount of larger oligoadenylates diminishes with increasing chain length (Kerr and Brown, 1978; Dougherty *et al.*, 1980). The oligoadenylates are elongated by the addition of adenylate residues. Diadenylates added to the enzyme are substrates for adenylate addition but two diadenylates do not become linked to each other (Justesen *et al.*, 1980b; Minks *et al.*, 1980).

$(2'-5')(A)_n$ synthetase was also reported to be capable of adding, in 2′–5′ linkage: (a) one or more adenylate residues or one nucleotide other than adenylate to a variety of compounds with 3′ terminal adenylate moieties, e.g. NAD, ADP-ribose, AppppA; (b) one nucleotide other than adenylate, to $(2'-5')(A)_n$; and (c) at least one adenylate residue to tRNA (Ball and White, 1979; Ferbus *et al.*, 1981).

The affinity of the enzyme for ATP is low; the K_m is about 2mM; (Minks *et al.*, 1979a; Justesen *et al.*, 1980a; Samanta *et al.*, 1980). The enzyme is maximally active when the concentration of double stranded RNA (w/v) is about one-half of that of the enzyme. In these conditions there is one enzyme molecule for every 80 base pair-long segment of the double stranded RNA (Samanta *et al.*, 1980). It is in line with this ratio that whereas double stranded RNA shorter than 30 base pairs does not activate the enzyme that longer than 65–80 base pairs causes maximal activation (Minks *et al.*, 1979c). Double stranded DNA or DNA–RNA hybrids cannot substitute for double stranded RNA in activating the enzyme (Ratner *et al.*, 1977; Ball and White, 1978).

$(2'-5')(A)_n$ synthetase was also isolated as a homogeneous protein from interferon-treated human (HeLa) cells (Yang *et al.*, 1981). It is somewhat smaller than the mouse enzyme (mol. wt 100 000 versus 105 000). The functional characteristics of the two enzymes are, however, very similar.

B RNase L: The Latent Endoribonuclease Activated by $(2'-5')(A)_n$

At present (but this might change, of course) the only well established biochemical function of $(2'-5')(A)_n$ is the activation of RNase L. The

$(2'-5')(A)_n$ has to be the trimer or longer to activate RNase L from Ehrlich ascites tumour, L929 or HeLa cells and the tetramer or longer to activate RNase L from rabbit reticulocyte lysates (Williams *et al.*, 1979a). Furthermore, to be able to activate either type of RNase L the oligoadenylates have to have triphosphate or diphosphate moieties at their 5′ termini (Martin *et al.*, 1979).

The activation of RNase L by $(2'-5')(A)_n$ is fully reversible: the addition of $(2'-5')(A)_n$ to a reaction mixture including latent RNase L results in activation of the enzyme. The removal of $(2'-5')(A)_n$ from the activated enzyme (e.g. by gel filtration) results in the reversion of the enzyme to the latent state. Readdition of $(2'-5')(A)_n$ to the now latent enzyme reactivates it (Slattery *et al.*, 1979).

The following results are consistent with the possibility that the activation of RNase L may involve the binding of $(2'-5')(A)_n$ to the enzyme: (1) whereas free $(2'-5')(A)_n$ passes through nitrocellulose filters, an RNase L preparation (partially purified from Ehrlich ascites tumour cells) can retain $(2'-5')(A)_n$ on nitrocellulose filters. (2) The agent retaining the oligoadenylates copurifies with RNase L during both ion exchange chromatography and gel filtration. (3) The treatment of RNase L with *N*-ethylmaleimide abolishes both its activatability by $(2'-5')(A)_n$ and its ability to retain these compounds on a nitrocellulose filter (Slattery *et al.*, 1980).

The molecular weight of RNase L is 185 000 as estimated by gel filtration. The activation of the enzyme does not seem to result in a large size change. This and other data make it unlikely that the activation should involve the binding or the release of a protein (Slattery *et al.*, 1979).

RNase L was partially (about 1000-fold) purified from an extract of Ehrlich ascites tumour cells by differential precipitation with ammonium sulphate and ion exchange chromatography (Floyd-Smith *et al.*, 1981; see also Schmidt *et al.*, 1978; Chernajovsky *et al.*, 1979). Most of the contaminating (i.e. $(2'-5')(A)_n$ independent) nucleases are removed in the course of this purification (Floyd-Smith *et al.*, 1981).

The early studies with unfractionated extracts from interferon-treated Ehrlich ascites tumour cells indicated that RNase L, if activated by $(2'-5')(A)_n$, cleaves various single stranded viral RNAs, cellular messenger RNAs (from both interferon-treated and control cells) and ribosomal RNAs at widely different rates. Double stranded RNAs are, however, not cleaved (Ratner *et al.*, 1977).

Recent experiments revealed that out of the four common homopolyribonucleotides (poly U, poly A, poly C and poly G) the RNase L purified from Ehrlich ascites tumour cells if activated by $(2'-5')(A)_n$ cleaves only poly U (Floyd-Smith *et al.*, 1981). Other studies with purified RNase L as well as with unfractionated rabbit reticulocyte lysates and crude extracts from mouse (Krebs ascites) cells and human (Daudi lymphoblastoid) cells indicate that in natural viral RNAs activated RNase L cleaves predominantly at the 3′ side of UA, UG, and UU sequences yielding 3′ phosphate terminated products (Floyd-Smith *et al.*, 1981; Wreschner *et al.*, 1981b). In single stranded RNA molecules with well defined secondary structures RNase L cleavages occur only in not hydrogen bonded, single stranded regions. The fact that the enzyme can efficiently cleave single stranded RNA at the 3′ side of at least three dinucleotides out of the 16 possible is consistent with the earlier findings revealing that RNase L is not specific for viral RNA (Ratner *et al.*, 1977).

It is curious that (1) the most preferred cleavage sites by activated RNase L include uridylate residues and (2) the activator of RNase L, $(2'\text{-}5')(A)_n$ consists of nucleotides complementary to uridylate. Whether or not direct U to A pairing occurs during cleavage by RNase L remains to be seen.

C (2′–5′) Phosphodiesterase Degrading $(2'\text{-}5')(A)_n$

In consequence of its unusual (2′–5′) phosphodiester linkages $(2'\text{-}5')(A)_n$ is resistant to many nucleases. However, $(2'\text{-}5')(A)_n$ is degraded in extracts from various cells, e.g. L929, HeLa and mouse reticulocytes (Williams *et al.*, 1978; Minks *et al.*, 1979b; Schmidt *et al.*, 1979; Ball, 1980). An enzyme designated as (2′–5′) phosphodiesterase, cleaving (2′–5′) phosphodiester linkages more efficiently that (3′–5′) linkages was partially purified from L929 cells (Schmidt *et al.*, 1979). This degrades $(2'\text{-}5')(A)_n$ into ATP and AMP. The presence of phosphate at the 5′ terminus of the oligoadenylates does not affect the rate of cleavage by this enzyme whereas the presence of a phosphate at the 3′ end impairs the cleavage. These results suggest that the enzyme may attack the oligonucleotides starting at their 3′ end. (2′–5′) phosphodiesterase has an apparent molecular weight of 40 000. It can catalyse the cleavage of various substances including that of the CCA termini of transfer RNAs.

VI $(2'\text{-}5')(A)_n$ SYNTHETASE, RNase L AND (2′–5′) PHOSPHODIESTERASE: PRESENCE IN TISSUES AND CULTURED CELLS. EFFECTS OF INTERFERONS AND OTHER AGENTS ON THE LEVEL OF THE ENZYMES

$(2'\text{-}5')(A)_n$ synthetase was found in a variety of vertebrates (e.g. mouse, guinea pig, rabbit, dog and chick). In the mouse it was detected in several tissues, including spleen, lungs, brain, liver, bone marrow, intestinal mucosa and serum. It is also present in a large variety of cultured human, mouse, monkey and chick cells (Ball, 1981). Furthermore it was reported to be packaged into the virions of vesicular stomatitis virus and Moloney mouse leukaemia virus grown in interferon-treated cells (Wallach and Revel, 1980).

The level of the enzyme is increased in cells upon treatment with interferons. The extent of this induction varies greatly: it is up to 10 000-fold in chick cells and only 10-fold in HeLa cells. The induction of the enzyme requires RNA synthesis and protein synthesis (Minks *et al.*, 1979a). The amount of the messenger RNA for (2′–5′)$(A)_n$ synthetase is increased in cells treated with interferon as revealed by the translation of messenger RNAs from control and interferon-treated cells in *Xenopus* oocytes into active enzyme (Shulman and Revel, 1980).

No difference was detected in the patterns of (2′–5′)$(A)_n$ synthetase induction in L929 cells (as far as interferon concentration dependence, kinetics and maximal levels of enzyme induced are concerned) between pure mouse interferon-α, pure mouse interferon-β and a 1:1 mixture of the two interferons (Broeze *et al.*, 1981). The induction by an interferon-γ preparation in HeLa cells was reported to be slower than that by an interferon-α preparation (Baglioni and Maroney, 1980; Hovanessian *et al.*, 1980). Furthermore induction by interferon-α was more "direct" than that by the interferon-γ. Interferon-α could induce the formation of (2′–5′)$(A)_n$ synthetase mRNA even in the presence of an inhibitor of protein synthesis (cycloheximide) since, upon removal of the inhibitor (to allow the translation of the messenger RNA to take place) and addition of actinomycin (to block further RNA synthesis), (2′–5′)$(A)_n$ synthetase was formed in the cells. Interferon-γ did not induce the enzyme under the above conditions. Thus it is conceivable that interferon-γ has to induce first intermediary proteins which in turn can activate the transcription of (2′–5′)$(A)_n$ synthetase messenger RNA.

The kinetics of induction vary between different cells. In L929 cells the level of the enzyme starts to increase within 3–5 h after the beginning of the treatment with interferons and reaches maximal levels by about 15 h (Broeze *et al.*, 1981). In some cells (e.g. HeLa) the enzyme induced by interferon seems to be stable. Thus its level in HeLa cells treated with interferon remains elevated even after the interferon has been removed from the medium and the specific enzyme activity appears to decrease only in consequence of the dilution by cell growth (Minks *et al.*, 1979a). In other cells (e.g. quiescent human fibroblasts) the level of (2′–5′)$(A)_n$ synthetase increases to the maximum in 24 hours after the beginning of the exposure to interferons but thereafter (though the cells remain exposed to interferon) decreases in four days to a level close to that in control cells (Krishnan and Baglioni, 1981). Thus in these cells (2′–5′)$(A)_n$ synthetase seems to be unstable. At least some of the enzyme in these cells is released into the medium and the release cannot be accounted for by lysis of dead cells.

Even in HeLa cells in which the induced (2′–5′)$(A)_n$ synthetase appears to be stable a transient exposure of cells to interferons results only in a transient commitment to the synthesis of (2′–5′)(A)$_n$ mRNA. An experiment involving the addition of an inhibitor of RNA synthesis (cordycepin) together with interferon followed by the removal of interferon and thereafter at various times of the inhibitor of RNA synthesis revealed the following: if the inhibitor was not removed within 5–6 h after the removal of interferon no (2′–5′)(A)$_n$ synthetase was formed. This indicates that the commitment of the cells to the induction of (2′–5′)(A)$_n$ synthetase decreased within a few hours after the removal of interferon if RNA synthesis is blocked. This result makes it probable that the effects of the interaction of interferons with the cell receptors are transient and have to be repeated or maintained for the continual stimulation of the transcription of (at least some of) the genetic regions activated by interferon (Baglioni and Maroney, 1980). This conclusion is in line with the results indicating that induction of (2′–5′)(A)$_n$ synthetase is arrested a few hours after the addition of anti-interferon antiserum (Revel *et al.*, 1980).

Studies of the induction of new proteins (as yet unidentified) by interferon involving (1) labelling cells with radioactive amino acid for short periods at different times after the beginning of the exposure to interferon and (2) analysis of the labelled proteins by gel electrophoresis) revealed a further feature of the regulation of interferon induction: even in the continued presence of interferons the synthesis of several induced proteins is only transient and the time period in which a particular protein is synthesized at the maximal rate is not the same for all the induced proteins (Gupta *et al.*, 1981).

The level of (2′–5′)(A)$_n$ synthetase is affected by agents other than interferons. Thus in chick oviducts the enzyme level is low and remains low after treatment with diethylstilboestrol but increases greatly after withdrawal of diethylstilboestrol (Stark *et al.*, 1979). In human lymphoblastoid cells (Raji, Daudi) treatment with glucocorticoids boosts the level of (2′–5′)(A)$_n$ synthetase up to 30-fold (Krishnan and Baglioni, 1980). In rabbit reticulocytes and human lymphocytes the level is high and it remains to be seen whether or not this is a consequence of endogenous exposure of the cells to interferons (Hovanessian and Kerr, 1978).

The level of (2′–5′)(A)$_n$ synthetase is also high in some cultured cell lines even without treatment with interferons. This is the case with a human line (HEC-1) and the mouse line (Kbalb) (Verhaegen *et al.*, 1980; Hovanessian *et al.*, 1981). The high level of (2′–5′)(A)$_n$ synthetase in the cells of the Kbalb line is a consequence of a constitutive production of interferon in an amount sufficient for boosting (2′–5′)(A)$_n$ synthetase formation. This conclusion is based on the finding that upon treatment of the cells with an antiserum to interferon for several weeks their level of (2′–5′)(A)$_n$ synthetase drops greatly (Hovanessian *et al.*, 1981).

In cells of MRC5, a human line, the level of the enzyme was reported to be below the level of detectability with or without interferon treatment (Meurs *et al.*, 1981).

The level of RNase L seems to be affected only slightly if at all by treatment with interferons (Schmidt *et al.*, 1978; Ratner, 1979). The constitutive level of this enzyme varies greatly in different mouse and human cells. In a transformed mouse line (NIH3T3) the RNase L activity was reported to be below the detectable level (Czarniecki *et al.*, 1981; Baglioni, personal communication). It is noteworthy that though interferon does induce $(2'–5')(A)_n$ synthetase in cells of this line, it does not impair in them the replication of either vesicular stomatitis virus or encephalomyocarditis virus.

The level of (2′–5′) phosphodiesterase is increased in L cells about threefold upon treatment with interferon (Schmidt *et al.*, 1979). In other cells, however, the level is unaffected by this treatment. The exposure of mouse spleen lymphocytes to concanavalin A was reported to boost the (2′–5′) phosphodiesterase level 5–6-fold. It is conceivable (see a later section) that this boost may be relevant to the mitogenic action of concanavalin A (Kimchi *et al.*, 1979a, 1981).

VII THE $(2'–5')(A)_n$ SYNTHETASE-RNase L PATHWAY IN INTACT CELLS

As described in earlier sections this pathway was discovered in experiments with *in vitro* systems. The definitive establishment of the function of the pathway *in vivo* may require cell mutants different from the wild type only in being defective or conditionally defective in one or the other of the two enzymes of the pathway. Such mutants are not available at present. However, numerous results obtained in experiments with intact cells are consistent with the assumption that this pathway is functioning *in vivo* and is mediating at least some of the antiviral activities of interferons.

A Accelerated Degradation of RNA in Interferon-treated, Reovirus-infected cells

The replication of reovirus in mouse L929 cells is inhibited by interferon and reovirus messenger RNAs are degraded faster in interferon-treated cells than in control cells. Thus in cells treated with interferon in which the reovirus yield is diminished by 80% the half-life of reovirus messenger RNA is 5·3 h whereas in control cells it is 12·3 h (Lengyel *et al.*, 1980).

Reovirus subviral particles (see the section on the inhibition of reovirus replication by interferon) isolated from cells which had been treated with interferon, when tested in a reaction mixture including ATP, reveal an endonuclease activity associated with the particles. However, subviral particles isolated from infected control cells, when tested under analogous conditions, appear to be free of nuclease (Galster and Lengyel, 1976). It remains to be shown, however, whether or not the endonuclease associated with the subviral particles from interferon-treated cells is RNase L, activated by $(2'\text{-}5')(A)_n$, which in turn is synthesized by $(2'\text{-}5')(A)_n$ synthetase that is bound to and is activated by the double stranded reo RNA in the particle.

The patterns of ribosomal RNA cleavage in intact interferon-treated (but not in control) cells infected with encephalomyocarditis virus overlap with those obtained on incubation of ribosomes in L cell extracts supplemented with $(2'\text{-}5')(A)_n$. This similarity in cleavage patterns may indicate that RNase L is active in such interferon-treated virus infected cells (Wreschner *et al.*, 1981a).

B Double Stranded RNA Enhances $(2'\text{-}5')(A)_n$ Formation and RNA Degradation in Interferon-treated Cells

The amount of $(2'\text{-}5')(A)_n$ in cells can be assayed by a binding competition assay involving labelled $(2'\text{-}5')(A)_n$ and a partially purified preparation of RNase L as a binding agent: the decrease in the binding of labelled $(2'\text{-}5')(A)_n$ is proportional to the amount of $(2'\text{-}5')(A)_n$ extracted from the cells (Knight *et al.*, 1980; Silverman *et al.*, 1981). Using this and other assays it was established that double stranded RNA (poly (I): poly (C)) added to intact interferon-treated (but not control) HeLa cells causes an increase in the level of $(2'\text{-}5')(A)_n$ and an enhancement of messenger RNA cleavage and polysome degradation (Nilsen *et al.*, 1981a).

C $(2'\text{-}5')(A)_n$ Accelerates RNA Cleavage and Inhibits Protein Synthesis and Virus Replication in Cells

The uptake of $(2'\text{-}5')(A)_n$ into intact cells can be facilitated by either permeabilizing the cells by treatment with a hypertonic solution or by using a $CaCl_2$ precipitation method (Williams and Kerr, 1978a; Hovanessian *et al.*, 1979). Using one or the other of these procedures it was established that $(2'\text{-}5')(A)_n$ added to hamster, mouse or monkey cells causes an enhancement of endonuclease activity concurrently with an inhibition of protein synthesis. Furthermore the addition of $(2'\text{-}5')(A)_n$ to virus infected cells results in a decrease of virus production (Williams and Kerr, 1978; Hovanessian *et al.*, 1979; Williams *et al.*, 1979b; Hovanessian and Wood, 1980).

D The level of $(2'–5')(A)_n$ in Intact Cells Increases upon Treatment with Interferon and Subsequent Infection with Encephalomyocarditis Virus

Experiments involving the binding competition assay revealed that the level of $(2'–5')(A)_n$ is at least 25-fold higher in cells treated with interferon and infected with encephalomyocarditis virus than in corresponding control cells. The interferon treatment alone or virus infection alone cause a much smaller increase in $(2'–5')(A)_n$ level (Williams *et al.*, 1979a; Knight *et al.*, 1980).

The replication of encephalomyocarditis virus and vesicular stomatitis virus is not impaired by interferon in a mouse cell line NIH3T3, chronically infected with Moloney murine leukaemia virus. Though the level of $(2'–5')(A)_n$ synthetase is enhanced in the cells of this line by treatment with interferons, that of RNase L remains below the level of detection (Czarniecki *et al.*, 1981). These observations are in line with the assumption that the $(2'–5')(A)_n$ synthetase RNase-L pathway is one of the mediators of interferon action.

E Interferon Action and the $(2'–5')(A)_n$ Synthetase-RNase L Pathway: Real or Apparent Anomalies

The picture is complicated, however, by observations on various cell lines. Thus, for example, it was reported that cells of the human HEC-1 and the mouse Kbalb line have high levels of $(2'–5')(A)_n$ synthetase (and apparently normal RNase L activity) and still are not in the antiviral state. Of these two lines Kbalb is (and HEC-1 is not) converted to the antiviral state by treatment with added interferons (Verhaegen *et al.*, 1980; Hovanessian *et al.*, 1981). Furthermore cells of the mouse MRC-5 line are low in $(2'–5')(A)_n$ synthetase activity even after treatment with interferon though the treatment does convert the cells into the antiviral state (Meurs *et al.*, 1981).

The resolution of these anomalies may require, among others, tests of the *in vivo* $(2'–5')(A)_n$ levels in these cells after treatment with interferon and virus infection. This is the case because these levels may determine if RNase L becomes activated and because the levels may be affected by agents other than $(2'–5')(A)_n$ synthetase, e.g. by various nucleases (including (2′–5′) phosphodiesterase) degrading $(2'–5')(A)_n$.

Moreover it has to be kept in mind that the $(2'–5')(A)_n$ synthetase–RNase L pathway is most probably only one of several mediators of the antiviral (and other) activities of interferons (Lengyel *et al.*, 1981; Maheshwari *et al.*, 1980; Kahana *et al.*, 1981). The impairment of the replication of a particular virus thus might require the functioning of particular mediators. Consequently in the cells showing the anomalous behaviour interferon mediators other than the $(2'–5')(A)_n$ synthetase-RNase L pathway might also be affected and this might perhaps be the basis of the anomalous behaviour.

The validity of these considerations seems to be supported by the characteristics of two cell lines. One of these is the NIH3T3 line (which as noted earlier is chronically infected with Moloney murine leukaemia virus and is low in, or lacking RNase L) in which the replication of vesicular stomatitis virus or of encephalomyocarditis virus is not impaired by interferon. In cells of this line, however, the interferon treatment does block the replication of Moloney murine leukaemia virus (Czarniecki *et al.*, 1981).

The second line in question is an undifferentiated mouse embryonal carcinoma line. It was reported that in cells of this line the interferon treatment enhances the level of $(2'\text{–}5')(A)_n$ synthetase (and presumably thereby that of the whole pathway). However, the treatment does not increase the level of another enzyme (a double stranded RNA activatable protein kinase) whose level is enhanced by interferons in several other types of cells. In cells of this line the treatment with interferon does not block the replication of vesicular stomatitis virus though it impairs that of encephalomyocarditis virus (Nilsen *et al.*, 1980b).

VIII WHY IS DOUBLE STRANDED RNA INVOLVED IN THE FUNCTIONING OF THE INTERFERON SYSTEM?

The $(2'\text{–}5')(A)_n$ synthetase–RNase L pathway is only one of the processes of the interferon system affected by double stranded RNA. Double stranded RNA is also an activator of another interferon-induced enzyme, a protein kinase (Lebleu *et al.*, 1976; Roberts *et al.*, 1976; Zilberstein *et al.*, 1976). If activated, this protein kinase phosphorylates and thereby inactivates the peptide chain initiation factor eIF-2 and thus inhibits protein synthesis (Farrell *et al.*, 1978; Sen *et al.*, 1978; Samuel, 1979; Kimchi *et al.*, 1979b). Furthermore, as noted earlier, double stranded RNA (viral or synthetic) induces the synthesis of interferons (Field *et al.*, 1967; Tytell *et al.*, 1967). Actually, a single molecule of double stranded RNA (in a defective interfering particle of a mutant vesicular stomatitis virus DI-011) per chick embryo cell was reported to be an efficient inducer of interferon synthesis (Marcus and Sekellick, 1977).

It is assumed that double stranded RNA became such an important modulator of the interferon system because (a) it may be formed as an intermediate, or side product in the replication of various viruses and thus (b) it may serve in the cell as a signal revealing the presence of certain types of replicating viruses.

Though these assumptions are reasonable they have to be tested for each virus. This is the case since in no type of virus can it be taken for granted that double stranded RNA of the required size for serving as a modulator of the interferon system is formed during replication, and even if it is, that it is available to serve as such a modulator.

Thus, in the case of viruses with a double stranded RNA genome (e.g. reovirus), the double stranded RNA is thought to be formed inside of a protein-coated particle (Joklik, 1974). Nevertheless reovirions were found to be able to substitute for free double stranded RNA in activating the (2′–5′)$(A)_n$ synthetase–RNase L pathway in an extract from interferon-treated cells (Lengyel *et al.*, 1980). However, the reovirions are only 4% as efficient on a "per milligram of double stranded RNA" basis as free double stranded RNA. Moreover, reovirions treated with RNase III (an enzyme specific for double stranded RNA cleavage), under conditions in which most free double stranded RNA but little or no double stranded RNA in virions was cleaved were no longer able to activate the pathway. This suggests that double stranded RNA on the surface of reovirions may be responsible for the activation of the (2′–5′)$(A)_n$ synthetase–RNase L system. The nature (viral or cellular) of this double stranded RNA on the virion surface has not been identified.

It is certain that the replication of single stranded RNA viruses requires the formation of complementary RNA strands. However, the formation of such complementary strands may only require the transient existence during replication of short double stranded stretches comprised of a segment of the template RNA strand and the complementary segment of the nascent RNA. Thus, to show that viral RNA extracted from cells infected with a single stranded RNA virus contains double stranded RNA is insufficient. This is because long double stranded RNA detected after the isolation of viral RNA may be an artefact formed *in vitro* by an association of complementary RNA strands only after removal of protein associated with the replicative RNA complexes (Borst and Weissmann, 1965). What has to be demonstrated is that during viral RNA replication in intact cells, double stranded RNA stretches are present which are sufficiently long to activate (2′–5′)$(A)_n$ synthetase (or protein kinase or induce interferon formation).

Recent experiments seem to indicate that one single stranded RNA virus (encephalomyocarditis virus) does generate stretches of double stranded RNA of sufficient length during replication (Nilsen and Baglioni, 1979). They revealed that a cellular fraction (not de-proteinized) from encephalomyocarditis virus infected HeLa cells (but not from uninfected cells) can activate the (2′–5′)$(A)_n$ synthetase-RNase L pathway in an extract of interferon-treated cells. It is in line with this observation that a cross-linking agent (4 aminoethyl-4,5,8-trimethyl psoralen, reported to be specific for double stranded RNA) did cross-link nascent viral RNA strands to template viral RNA strands in intact encephalomyocarditis virus infected HeLa cells (Nilsen *et al.*, 1981b).

Double stranded viral RNA was also found in RNA extracted from cells infected with a DNA virus: vaccinia (Colby and Duesberg, 1969; Boone *et al.*, 1979). It was not established, however, if the double stranded RNA exists as such *in vivo* or is formed only after RNA extraction.

More definitive approaches than those used in the above experiments are available and should be used in the future for testing if a virus activates in interferon-treated cells the (2′–5′)$(A)_n$ synthetase–RNase L pathway. These are based on (a) the determination of the endogenous level of the nuclease activator (2′–5′)$(A)_n$ and (b) the comparison of the rate of turnover of viral RNA in interferon-treated and control cells. These approaches should clearly establish which virus does, and which does not, generate appropriate double stranded RNA for the activation of the pathway in question.

IX WHY IS DOUBLE STRANDED RNA NEEDED TO ACTIVATE THE (2′–5′)$(A)_n$ SYNTHETASE–RNase L PATHWAY?

It is puzzling why double stranded RNA, which is involved in the induction of interferon, is also required for the activation of at least some of the interferon-induced enzymes. This complexity might be rationalized in the following hypothesis: virus infection (perhaps if accompanied by the formation of some double stranded RNA) may result in the synthesis of interferons in the infected cells and the secretion and spreading of these interferons in the organism. In the cells exposed to interferons the synthesis of (2′–5′)$(A)_n$ synthetase and of double stranded RNA activatable protein kinase are induced. Since both of these enzymes are latent, they do not impair the metabolism of uninfected cells. However, when the cells, previously exposed to interferons, become infected with virus, this may result in the formation of some double stranded RNA and thereby the activation of the two enzyme systems. This in turn impairs the metabolism of the virus-infected cells, and thereby inhibits virus replication. Thus, ultimately this complex control system may contribute to the localization of viral infection (Kerr *et al.*, 1974; Ratner *et al.*, 1977).

In vitro the (2′–5′)$(A)_n$ synthetase–RNase L system appears to cleave viral and host RNAs without discrimination. *In vivo*, however, at least in the case of some virus–cell systems (e.g. reovirus-L929 cells), viral protein synthesis is inhibited preferentially above host protein synthesis (Gupta *et al.*, 1974). An intriguing series of experiments *in vitro* reveals that, at least in principle, the double stranded RNA involved in activating the (2′–5′)$(A)_n$ synthetase–RNase L system, might make this system capable of such discrimination (Nilsen and Baglioni, 1979; Nilsen *et al.*, 1980a). For these experiments poly U was annealed to the poly A segment of a viral RNA (from vesicular stomatitis virus) resulting in a viral RNA in which a single stranded segment is covalently linked to a double stranded segment. In an extract from interferon-treated cells supplemented wtih ATP this viral RNA covalently bound to a double stranded RNA segment is degraded faster than an identical viral RNA not bound to double stranded RNA. This result is consistent with the possibility that in interferon-treated cells infected by an RNA virus the RNase L activity may be restricted to a region near to the partially double stranded replicative intermediate of the virus. Such a localization might be a consequence of (1) the localized synthesis of $(2'-5')(A)_n$ by the $(2'-5')(A)_n$ synthetase bound to the partially double stranded viral replicative intermediate and (2) the decrease in the concentration of $(2'-5')(A)_n$ away from its site of formation that is caused by cleavage by $(2'-5')$ phosphodiesterase. It is also conceivable, however, that RNase L may form a complex with $(2'-5')(A)_n$ synthetase and this might be the basis of the localization. It remains to be established if RNase L activity is localized *in vivo.*

X DOES THE $(2'-5')(A)_n$ SYNTHETASE–RNase L PATHWAY HAVE ANY FUNCTIONS THAT ARE UNRELATED TO THE ANTIVIRAL ACTIONS OF INTERFERONS OR EVEN TO INTERFERON ACTION?

Studies with highly purified interferon preparations established that interferons (and not only the impurities in interferon preparations) can inhibit the growth of cultured cells and mitogenesis induced in lymphocytes by mitogens (Kawakita *et al.,* 1978; De Maeyer-Guignard *et al.,* 1980). Experiments with mouse spleen lymphocytes revealed that not only interferons, but also exogenous $(2'-5')(A)_n$ can block mitogenesis induced by concanavalin A.

The primary effect of $(2'-5')(A)_n$ in inhibiting mitogenesis seems to be an impairment of the synthesis of many proteins including histones (Kimchi *et al.*, 1979a, 1981).

It should be noted that in the above experiments not $(2'-5')(A)_n$ (i.e. oligoadenylates with 5′ terminal triphosphates) were used, but $(2'-5')(A)_n$ "core", i.e. the product obtained by removing the 5′ triphosphate of $(2'-5')(A)_n$ with alkaline phosphatase. $(2'-5')(A)_n$ core does not activate RNase L *in vitro* and is only one-tenth as active as $(2'-5')(A)_n$ in inhibiting protein synthesis if added to permeabilized cells (Williams and Kerr, 1978). It has, however, an important advantage over $(2'-5')(A)_n$: it is taken up even by nonpermeabilized cells (Kimchi *et al.*, 1979a). $(2'-5')(A)_n$ core occurs in vivo and its level is enhanced in L929 cells upon treatment with interferon and infection with encephalomyocarditis virus (Knight *et al.*, 1980). The mechanism of action of $(2'-5')(A)_n$ core is unknown. It is conceivable that the compound might be activated in cells by phosphorylation to $(2'-5')(A)_n$ (i.e. $pppA(pA)_n$) or it might increase the level of endogenous $(2'-5')(A)_n$ by blocking (2′–5′) phosphodiesterase (Kimchi *et al.*, 1981). It is also conceivable that the compound is affecting agents other than RNase L, and is acting as is.

There are several observations in line with the possibility that $(2'-5')(A)_n$ might be among the agents controlling the rate of cell division. The treatment of lymphocytes with concanavalin A causes a several-fold increase in the level of (2′–5′) phosphodiesterase without affecting the level of $(2'-5')(A)_n$ synthetase. The level of (2′–5′) phosphodiesterase is three-fold higher in dividing cells than in confluent cells of a monkey cell line (AGMK). Serum starvation decreases whereas the addition of serum increases the level of the enzyme. Finally, the ratio of $(2'-5')(A)_n$ synthetase to (2′–5′) phosphodiesterase (that determines the level of $(2'-5')(A)_n$) is 10-fold lower in fast growing (AGMK) cells than in confluent cells (arrested in the G_0 phase by serum starvation) (Kimchi *et al.*, 1979a, 1981).

It remains to be established if the $(2'-5')(A)_n$ synthetase–RNase L pathway or either of the two enzymes involved has any functions seemingly unrelated to interferon action. There are several facts consistent with this possibility. The level of RNase L is little, if at all, affected by interferons. Furthermore, the level of $(2'-5')(A)_n$ synthetase is, as noted earlier, affected by agents other than interferons (e.g. oestrogen withdrawal, glucocorticoids) (Stark *et al.*, 1979; Krishnan and Baglioni, 1980).

Since the pathway, if activated, catalyses RNA cleavage it is reasonable to assume that a function possibly unrelated to interferon action would also consist of RNA cleavage, e.g. steps in processing of heterogeneous nuclear RNA, degradation of messenger RNA or ribosomal RNA. It may be relevant to note that heterogeneous nuclear RNA appears to contain essentially double stranded stretches (Jelinek and Darnell, 1972; Robertson *et al.*, 1977; Calvet and Pederson, 1979) and cellular RNA was reported to serve as a substitute for double stranded RNA (though a very inefficient one) in activating the $(2'-5')(A)_n$ synthetase–RNase L pathway (Revel *et al.*, 1980).

Thus, it is conceivable that interferons are making use of enzymes which in the absence of interferons are utilized for unrelated purposes, and interferon action is based in part on an increased production of such enzymes. It is also possible, however, that the scope of interferon action is wider than imagined at present and purposes seemingly unrelated fall within this scope.

XI CONCLUSIONS

The (2′–5′)$(A)_n$ synthetase–RNase L pathway was discovered in experiments with extracts from interferon-treated cells. It consists of two steps (see Fig. 1). (2′–5′)$(A)_n$ synthetase has been purified to homogeneity from both mouse and human cells and the products, stoichiometry, equilibrium and optimal conditions for the reaction it catalyses have been determined. RNase L has been purified about 1000-fold, to a state in which it is essentially free of (2′–5′)$(A)_n$ independent nuclease activity. The activation of the latent enzyme by (2′–5′)$(A)_n$ is reversible. The activated RNase L cleaves single stranded RNA. The preferred cleavage sites are at the 3′ side of UA, UG and UU sequences. The products have 3′ terminal phosphate residues. The treatment of cells with interferons induces the formation of (2′–5′)$(A)_n$ synthetase by an as yet undetermined mechanism. The same treatment affects the level of RNase L if at all, only slightly. There are a large variety of data consistent with the view that this pathway is among the mediators of the antiviral activity of interferons. Furthermore (2′–5′)$(A)_n$ may also be among the agents controlling cell division.

XII ACKNOWLEDGEMENTS

Studies in the author's laboratory were supported by research grants AI-12320 and CA16038 from the NIH USPHS.

XIII REFERENCES

Baglioni, C. and Maroney, P. (1980). *J. biol. Chem.* **255**, 8390–8393.
Baglioni, C., Minks, M. A. and Maroney, P. A. (1978). *Nature, Lond.* **273**, 684–687.
Ball, L. A. (1980). *Ann. N.Y. Acad. Sci.* **350**, 486–496.
Ball, L. A. (1981). *In* "The Enzymes" (Ed. P. D. Boyer) Vol. 15. In press.
Ball, L. A. and White, C. N. (1978). *Proc. natn. Acad. Sci. U.S.A.* **75**, 1167–1171.
Ball, L. A. and White, C. N. (1978). *In* "Regulation of Macromolecular Synthesis by Low Molecular Weight Mediators" (Eds E. Koch and D. Richter) 303–317. Academic Press, New York.
Bialy, H. S. and Colby, C. (1972). *J. Virol.* **9**, 286–289.
Boone, R. F., Parr, R. P. and Moss, B. (1979). *J. Virol.* **30** 365–374.
Borst, P. and Weissmann, C. (1965). *Proc. natn. Acad. Sci. U.S.A.* **54**, 982–987.
Broeze, R., Dougherty, J. P., Pichon, J., Jayaram, B. M. and Lengyel, P. (1981). *J. Interferon Res.* **1**, 191–201.
Brown, G. E., Lebleu, B., Kawakita, M., Shaila, S., Sen, G. C. and Lengyel, P. (1976). *Biochem. biophys. Res. Commun.* **69**, 114–122.
Calvet, J. P. and Pederson, T. (1979). *Proc. natn. Acad. Sci. U.S.A.* **76**, 755–759.

Chernajovsky, Y., Kimchi, A., Schmidt, A., Zilberstein, A. and Revel, M. (1979). *Eur. J. Biochem.* **96**, 35–41.
Clemens, M. J. and Williams, B. R. G. (1978). *Cell* **13**, 565–572.
Colby, C. and Duesberg, P. H. (1969). *Nature, Lond.* **222**, 940–944.
Czarniecki, C. W., Sreevalsan, T., Friedman, R. M. and Panet, A. (1981). *J. Virol.* **37**, 827–831.
DeClercq, E., Stewart, W. E., II, and De Somer, P. (1972). *Immunology* **6**, 344–347.
DeMaeyer-Guignard, J., DeMaeyer, E., Tovey, M. G. and Gresser, I. (1980). *Ann. N.Y. Acad. Sci.* **350**, 347–353.
Doornbos, J., Den Hartog, J. A. J., Boom, J. H. v. and Altona, C. (1981). *Eur. J. Biochem.* **116**, 403–412.
Dougherty, J. P., Samanta, H., Farrell, P. J. and Lengyel, P. (1980). *J. biol. Chem.* **255**, 3813–3816.
Ehrenfeld, E. and Hunt, T. (1971). *Proc. natn. Acad. Sci. U.S.A.* **68**, 1075–1078.
Farrell, P. J., Sen, G. C., Dubois, M. F., Ratner, L., Slattery, E. and Lengyel, P. (1978). *Proc. natn. Acad. Sci. U.S.A.* **75**, 5893–5897.
Ferbus, D., Justesen, J., Besançon, F. and Thang, M. N. (1981). *Biochem. biophys. Res. Commun.* **100**, 847–856.
Field, A. K., Tytell, A. A., Lampson, G. P. and Hilleman, M. R. (1967). *Proc. natn. Acad. Sci. U.S.A.* **58**, 1004–1010.
Floyd-Smith, G., Slattery, E. and Lengyel, P. (1981). *Science, N.Y.* **212**, 1030–1032.
Galster, R. L. and Lengyel, P. (1976). *Nucl. Acids Res.* **3**, 581–598.
Gravell, M. and Cromeans, T. L. (1972). *Virology* **50**, 916–919.
Graziadei, W. D. III, Roy, D., Konigsberg, W. and Lengyel, P. (1973). *Archs Biochem. Biophys.* **158**, 266–275.
Gupta, S. L., Graziadei, W. D. III, Weideli, H., Sopori, M. L. and Lengyel, P. (1974). *Virology* **57**, 49–63.
Gupta, S. L., Rubin, B. Y. and Holmes, S. L. (1981). *Virology* **111**, 331–340.
Hovanessian, A. G. and Kerr, I. M. (1978). *Eur. J. Biochem.* **84**, 149–159.
Hovanessian, A. G. and Kerr, I. M. (1979). *Eur. J. Biochem.* **93**, 515–526.
Hovanessian, A. G. and Ward, J. N. (1980). *Virology* **101**, 81–90.
Hovanessian, A. G., Brown, R. E. and Kerr, I. (1977). *Nature, Lond.* **268**, 532–540.
Hovanessian, A. G., Wood, J., Meurs, E. and Montagnier, L. (1979). *Proc. natn. Acad. Sci. U.S.A.* **76**, 3261–3265.
Hovanessian, A. G., LaBonnardiere, C. and Falcoff, E. (1980). *J. Interferon Res.* **1**, 125–135.
Hovanessian, A. G., Meurs, E. and Montagnier, J. (1981). *J. Interferon Res.* **1**, 179–190.
Jelinek, W. and Darnell, J. E. (1972). *Proc. natn. Acad. Sci. U.S.A.* **69**, 2537–2541.
Joklik, W. K. (1974). *In* "Comprehensive Virology" (Eds H. Fraenkel-Conrat and R. R. Wagner) Vol. 2, 231–339. Plenum Press, New York and London.
Justesen, J., Ferbus, D. and Thang, M. N. (1980a). *Ann. N.Y. Acad. Sci.* **350**, 510–521.
Justesen, J., Ferbus, D. and Thang, M. N. (1980b). *Proc. natn. Acad. Sci. U.S.A.* **77**, 9618–9622.
Kahana, C., Yakobson, E., Revel, M. and Groner, Y. (1981). *Virology* **112**, 109–118.
Kawakita, M. B., Cabrer, B., Taira, H., Rebello, M., Slattery, E., Weideli, H. and Lengyel, P. (1978). *J. biol. Chem.* **253**, 598–602.
Kerr, I. M. and Brown, R. E. (1978). *Proc. natn. Acad. Sci. U.S.A.* **75**, 256–260.
Kerr, I. M., Brown, R. E. and Ball, L. A. (1974). *Nature, Lond.* **250**, 57–59.

Kimchi, A., Shure, H. and Revel, M. (1979a). *Nature, Lond.* **282**, 849–851.
Kimchi, A., Zilberstein, A., Schmidt, A., Shulman, L. and Revel, M. (1979b). *J. biol. Chem.* **254**, 9846–9853.
Kimchi, A., Shure, H. and Revel, M. (1981). *Eur. J. Biochem.* **114**, 5–10.
Knight, M., Cayley, P. J., Silverman, R. H., Wreschner, D. H., Gilbert, C. S., Brown, R. E. and Kerr, I. M. (1980). *Nature, Lond.* **288**, 189–192.
Krishnan, I. and Baglioni, C. (1980). *Proc. natn. Acad. Sci. U.S.A.* **77**, 6506–6510.
Krishnan, I. and Baglioni, C. (1981). *Virology* **111**, 666–670.
Lebleu, B., Sen, G. C., Shaila, S., Cabrer, B. and Lengyel, P. (1976). *Proc. natn. Acad. Sci. U.S.A.* **73**, 3107–3111.
Lengyel, P. (1981). *In* "Eukaryotic Protein Synthesis" (Ed. R. Perez Bercoff). Plenum Press, New York and London. In press.
Lengyel, P., Desrosiers, R., Broeze, R., Slattery, E., Taira, H., Dougherty, J., Samanta, H., Pichon, J., Farrell, P., Ratner, L. and Sen, G. (1980). *In* "Microbiology-1980" (Ed. D. Schlessinger) 219–226. American Society for Microbiology.
Maheshwari, R. K., Banerjee, D. K., Waechter, C. J., Olden, K., and Friedman, R. M. (1980). *Nature, Lond.* **287**, 454–456.
Manders, F. K., Tilles, J. G. and Huang, A. S. (1972). *Virology* **49**, 573–581.
Marcus, P. and Sekellick, M. J. (1977). **266**, 815–819.
Marcus, P. I., Engelhardt, D. L., Hunt, J. M., Sekellick, M. J. (1971). *Science, N.Y.* **174**, 593–598.
Martin, E. M., Birdsall, N. J. M., Brown, R. E. and Kerr, I. M. (1979). *Eur. J. Biochem.* **95**, 295–307.
Meurs, E., Hovanessian, A. G. and Montagnier, L. (1981). *J. Interferon Res.* **1**, 219–232.
Minks, M. A., Benvin, S., Maroney, P. A. and Baglioni, C. (1979a). *J. biol. Chem.* **254**, 5058–5064.
Minks, M. A., Maroney, P. A. and Baglioni, C. (1979b). *Nucl. Acids Res.* **6**, 767–780.
Minks, M. A., West, D. K., Benvin, S. and Baglioni, C. (1979c). *J. biol. Chem.* **254**, 10180–10183.
Minks, M. A., Benvin, S. and Baglioni, C. (1980). *J. biol. Chem.* **255**, 5031–5035.
Nilsen, T. W. and Baglioni, C. (1979). *Proc. natn. Acad. Sci. U.S.A.* **76**, 2600–2604.
Nilsen, T. W., Weissmann, S. G. and Baglioni, C. (1980a). *Biochemistry* **19**, 5574–5579.
Nilsen, T. W., Wood, D. L. and Baglioni, C. (1980b). *Nature, Lond.* **286**, 178–180.
Nilsen, T. W., Maroney, P. A. and Baglioni, C. (1981a). *J. biol. Chem.* In press.
Nilsen, T. W., Wood, D. L. and Baglioni, C. (1981b). *Virology* **109**, 82–93.
Oxman, M. N. and Levine, M. J. (1971). *Proc. natn. Acad. Sci. U.S.A.* **68**, 299–302.
Ratner, L. (1979). Dissertation, Yale University.
Ratner, L., Sen, G. C., Brown, G. E., Lebleu, B., Kawakita, M., Cabrer, B., Slattery, E. and Lengyel, P. (1977). *Eur. J. Biochem.* **79**, 565–577.
Ratner, L., Wiegand, R., Farrell, P., Sen, G. C., Cabrer, B. and Lengyel, P. (1978). *Biochem. biophys. Res. Commun.* **81**, 947–957.
Revel, M., Kimchi, A., Shulman, L., Fradin, A., Shuster, R., Yakobson, E., Chernajovsky, Y., Schmidt, A., Shure, A. and Bendori, R. (1980). *Ann. N.Y. Acad. Sci.* **350**, 459–472.
Roberts, W. K., Hovanessian, A., Brown, R. E., Clemens, M. J. and Kerr, I. M. (1976). *Nature, Lond.* **264**, 477–480.
Robertson, H. D., Dickson, E. and Jelinek, W. (1977). *J. molec. Biol.* **115**, 571–589.

Samanta, H., Dougherty, J. P. and Lengyel, P. (1980). *J. biol. Chem.* **255**, 9807-9813.
Samuel, C. E. (1979). *Proc. natn. Acad. Sci. U.S.A.* **76**, 600-604.
Schmidt, A., Zilberstein, A., Shulman, L., Federman, P., Berissi, H. and Revel, M. (1978). *FEBS Lett.* **95**, 257-264.
Schmidt, A., Chernajovsky, Y., Shulman, L., Federman, P., Berissi, H. and Revel, M. (1979). *Proc. natn. Acad. Sci. U.S.A.* **76**, 4788-4792.
Sen, G. C., Lebleu, B., Brown, G. E., Rebello, M. A., Furuichi, Y., Morgan, M., Shatkin, A. J. and Lengyel, P. (1975). *Biochem. biophys. Res. Commun.* **65**, 427-434.
Sen, G. C., Lebleu, B., Brown, G. E., Kawakita, M., Slattery, E. and Lengyel, P. (1976). *Nature, Lond.* **264**, 370-373.
Sen, G. C., Taira, H. and Lengyel, P. (1978). *J. biol. Chem.* **253**, 5915-5921.
Shaila, S., Lebleu, B., Brown, G. E., Sen, G. C. and Lengyel, P. (1977). *J. gen. Virol.* **37**, 535-546.
Shulman, L. and Revel. M. (1980). *Nature, Lond.* **288**, 98-100.
Silverman, R. H., Wreschner, D. H., Gilbert, C. S. and Kerr, I. M. (1981). *Eur. J. Biochem.* **115**, 79-85.
Slattery, E., Ghosh, N., Samanta, H. and Lengyel, P. (1979). *Proc. natn. Acad. Sci. U.S.A.* **76**, 4778-4782.
Slattery, E., Ghosh, N., Samanta, H. and Lengyel, P. (1980). *In* "Interferon: Properties and Clinical Uses" (Eds A. Khan and G. L. Dorn) 521-528. Wadley Institutes of Molecular Medicine.
Stark, G. R., Dower, W. J., Schimke, R. T., Brown, R. E. and Kerr, I. M. (1979). *Nature, Lond.* **278**, 471-473.
Stewart, W. E., II (1979). "The Interferon System." Springer-Verlag, New York.
Stewart, W. E., II, DeClercq, E., Billiau, A., Desmyter, J. and DeSomer, P. (1972). *Proc. natn. Acad. Sci. U.S.A.* **69**, 1851-1854.
Taylor-Papadimitriou, J. (1980). *In* "Interferon 1980 Volume 2" (Ed. I. Gresser), 13-42. Academic Press, London and New York.
Tytell, A. A., Lampson, G. P., Field, A. U. and Hilleman, R. M. (1967). *Proc. natn. Acad. Sci. U.S.A.* **58**, 1719-1722.
Verhaegen, M., Divizia, M., Vandenbussche, P., Kuwata, T. and Content, J. (1980). *Proc. natn. Acad. Sci. U.S.A.* **77**, 4479-4483.
Vilček, J., Gresser, I. and Merigan, T. C. (Eds) (1980). "Regulatory Function of Interferons" 1-641. *Ann. N.Y. Acad. Sci.* **350**.
Wallach, D. and Revel, M. (1980). *Nature, Lond.* **287**, 68-70.
Wiebe, M. E. and Joklik, W. K. (1975). *Virology* **66**, 229-240.
Williams, B. R. G. and Kerr, I. M. (1978). *Nature, Lond.* **276**, 88-90.
Williams, B. R. G., Kerr, I. M., Gilbert, C. S., White, C. N. and Ball, L. A. (1978). *Eur. J. Biochem.* **92**, 455-462.
Williams, B. R. G., Golgher, R. R., Brown, R. E., Gilbert, C. S. and Kerr, I. M. (1979a). *Nature, Lond.* **282**, 582-586.
Williams, B. R. G., Golgher, R. R. and Kerr, I. M. (1979b). *FEBS Lett.* **105**, 47-52.
Wreschner, D. H., James, T. C., Silverman, R. H. and Kerr, I. M. (1981a). *Nucl. Acids Res.* **9**, 1571-1581.
Wreschner, D. H., McCauley, J. W., Skehel, J. J. and Kerr, I. M. (1981b). *Nature, Lond.* **289**, 414-417.
Yang, K., Samanta, H., Dougherty, J., Jayaram, B., Broeze, R. and Lengyel, P. (1981). *J. biol. Chem.* **256**, 9324-9328.
Zilberstein, A., Federman, P., Shulman, L. and Revel, M. (1976). *FEBS Lett.* **68**, 119-124.

The Cloning of Interferon and Other Mistakes

CHARLES WEISSMANN

Institut für Molekularbiologie I, Universität Zürich, Zürich, Switzerland

I ON THE MERITS OF STROLLING

In the summer of 1977 at a Gordon Conference I took my annual walk with Peter Lengyel, and, as he described the complexities of the mode of action of mouse interferon and of the control of its expression, it became evident that cloning of the chromosomal interferon gene would lead to a wealth of information unattainable by any other means. Moreover, the undertaking was a challenge, since pure interferon was extremely hard to come by, its structure was unknown and would probably not be elucidated for years to come, no good antibodies to IFN were known to be available, and the mRNA was presumably present at a very low level. However, as Peter explained to me, there did exist a very sensitive assay for interferon mRNA: the injection of about 50 ng of poly (A) RNA from interferon-producing cells into each of a dozen *Xenopus* oocytes led to synthesis (Reynolds *et al.*, 1975) of easily measurable amounts of interferon. It occurred to me that an assay for cloned interferon cDNA might be based on a hybridization procedure in connection with this interferon mRNA assay (see Figs 1 and 2). Assume you already possess an interferon cDNA clone, and that you fix it to a solid support such as a Millipore filter. If this filter is annealed with poly (A) RNA containing IFN mRNA and then washed, you would expect it to retain the IFN mRNA, but none of the other mRNAs. If the filter is subsequently heated in water, the RNA–DNA hybrids will be denatured and the IFN mRNA can be washed off and assayed in the oocyte test. If any other hybrid cDNA is attached to the filter, some other mRNA will be bound and subsequently recovered, and the oocyte assay will be negative for interferon. This procedure would thus allow the identification of an IFN cDNA plasmid (or, with appropriate modifications, other plasmids of interest, as was shown a year later by Harpold *et al.* (1978) for rat growth hormone) but it is so time-consuming and labour intensive that the screening of thousands or of even only hundreds of clones would be an overwhelming task. However, if one were to examine the plasmid DNA from pools of, say, 1000 clones at a time, then one could rapidly screen 10 000 clones, identify a positive group, and then rescreen the clones of that group in subgroups of 100 each. This procedure, known in genetics as subculture cloning, would be repeated with decreasing group size, until the interferon cDNA clone was identified. Peter had an additional suggestion, namely that one make use of the fact that only induced, but not non-induced cells produce interferon mRNA. Thus, one could, for example, make cDNA from noninduced cells, hybridize an excess of it with mRNA from induced cells and separate the nonhybridized RNA—which should consist mainly of mRNA present in induced but not in noninduced cells. This partially purified mRNA could then be used as starting material for the cloning, or as the basis for a hybridization probe. Whatever the approach, Peter and I agreed that the project was feasible and at the end of our stroll we decided to undertake it. In the autumn of 1977 Peter Lengyel sent us partially purified poly (A) mRNA from interferon-producing mouse Ehrlich ascites tumour cells and Peter Curtis, who had previously purified the 15 S β-globin mRNA precursor and done quite a lot of cDNA cloning, undertook further purification by the hybridization approach Lengyel had suggested. However, the first attempts did not appear very promising and I decided that our time would be better spent preparing a clone bank and searching through it by the hybridization–translation approach. The in itself simple task of cloning mouse cDNA was fraught with man-made difficulties, because the restrictions on work with recombinant DNA were in full bloom. Shot-gun cloning of DNA from virus-infected eukaryotic cells required so-called P4 conditions (I hope by the time this article is published most readers will no longer know what this means), which were not available to me in Zürich. At this point I must digress and relate a fateful development that was occurring while this work was underway.

II ENTER BIOGEN

A year earlier, in February 1977, I had been visited by Ray Schäfer, a former Research Director of Inco, and Dan Adams, a lawyer and investment banker, also of Inco. They were touring Europe and interviewing the local talent as to its interest in participating in the commercialization of recombinant DNA technology, along the lines pioneered by Herb Boyer and his company Genentech. I was decidedly uninterested and limited my efforts to providing the Inco emissaries with some further addresses. However, early in 1978 the duo was back again and this time captured my interest. They proposed to create a company, Biogen, which would be advised by a Scientific Board consisting of (as they put it) the most prominent molecular biologists in Europe and in addition, Wally Gilbert and Phil Sharp. As Wally was one of the molecular biologists whom I admired unreservedly, both for his superb mind and his capacity for promoting achievement, it seemed to me that whatever drawbacks my involvement with a commercial venture might bring, an association with Wally would be a redeeming feature. I was thus receptive to an invitation to what was described as "First European Microbiology Conference", but in fact constituted a meeting of the members designate of the Biogen Scientific Board: Wally Gilbert (Harvard University), Brian Hartley (Imperial College), Peter-Hans Hofschneider (Max-Planck Institute, München), Philippe Kourilsky (Institut Pasteur, Paris), Bernard Mach (Institute of Microbiology, University of Geneva), Ken Murray (University of Edinburgh), Ray Schäfer (Inco), Heinz Schaller (University of Heidelberg), Phil Sharp (MIT, Boston) and myself—listed alphabetically and not necessarily by merit. (About a year later Kourilsky had to leave the group because of his commitments to the Pasteur Institute, and I brought in Walter Fiers from Ghent, an old friend and competitor, to replace him.)

We were received in Geneva in surroundings of unmatched luxury (unmatched above all in Biogen meetings subsequent to our signing up) and were pampered from breakfast to bedtime. Our discussions revolved around the possible structure of the company, as well as the feasibility and profitability of a project list I had drawn up and to which some additional possibilities had been added. To the delight of the organizers I revealed that our laboratory was already working on the cloning of mouse interferon and that I would be prepared to extend our efforts to the human system. We disbanded, agreeing to meet some weeks later and communicate our decision as to whether we would go ahead to form a company. At this meeting in Paris, on March 25–27, 1978, we were amazed to discover that all of us had decided to join Biogen. Considerable time was devoted to discussing the structure of the proposed company. Briefly, the Scientific

Board would provide the scientific direction and members of the Board would undertake projects in their laboratories according to their possibilities. Except for a modest *per diem* fee for attending meetings, all services were to be compensated by shares—both for serving on the board, and for undertaking and accomplishing determined research goals. Indeed, the only expenses resulting to Biogen would be for supplies, support of postdoctorals and technicians, and overheads to the universities. The pay-off for the scientists (other than the occasional good meal and the annual January Board Meeting on a Caribbean island) would come about when the shares became negotiable, after seven years or upon "going public", whichever came first. The scientists stipulated that one third of the Directors would be chosen from the members of the Scientific Board, to ensure that the interests of the scientists were being represented at all levels. One such interest was to prevent a sell-out of the company to a large corporation; our major concern, however, was to conserve full freedom of publication and scientific communication, clearly a difficult position to reconcile with demands for patent protection and protection of know-how demanded by commercial partners. We eventually hammered out an arrangement which was to prove satisfactory to the scientists, reasonably so to Biogen but a source of occasional irritation to our future commercial partners. In essence, the scientists undertook to do their best to secure patent applications for all commercially useful achievements prior to publication, but they were not under constraint to secure Biogen's permission for publication. The decision on how to handle our scientific results, including the distribution of strains, thus became our responsibility, and I suppose each of us reacted according to his nature. Those of us who were naturally secretive or uncommunicative could continue to be so to the satisfaction of the commercial partners, while the extroverts would be essentially free to disseminate their own data to their hearts' desire. However, in these same hearts they had to know that a failure to safeguard patent applications or technical know-how might run counter to the interests of the company they were trying to create. There is no denying that a new motivation had appeared to diminish the flow of information, but I am not sure whether it was stronger than the all-pervading pre-existing motivation of being the first to discover and to out-do his colleagues and competitors. The scale of communication even in the "pre-commercial" days ranged from the absolute openness of Tom Maniatis, who provided his rivals with materials and methods that helped them compete with their benefactor, to the total secretiveness of colleagues working in the same building who interdicted their "postdocs" to talk to each other.

III YOU NEVER CAN TELL

The nascent Scientific Board officially commissioned me to clone human interferon cDNA as a Biogen project, and decided to support the mouse project as well, since I believed that a mouse interferon clone could be used to screen for a human clone by nonstringent colony hybridization (this assumption proved to be correct, inasmuch as we ultimately used human interferon cDNA to identify mouse clones). Brian Hartley arranged for the permission of the British Genetic Manipulation Advisory Group to clone the mouse cDNA in his C3 suite, which solved a major problem for us—the first benefit of the "Biogen network". Since our lab had no experience with induction and measurement of interferon and Peter Lengyel had no source of human interferon mRNA, I had to find a partner who would collaborate with us on the human interferon project. A quick survey of the literature had made it clear that the ideal partner would be Kari Cantell in Helsinki, who had transformed interferon from a laboratory curiosity into a potential clinical tool. Interferon, it should be realized, is produced only in minute quantities by virus-induced leukocytes; after a decade of improvements, 10^{10} cells incubated in 1 litre of medium were brought to produce about 50×10^6 units, that is, about 250 μg of interferon. Kari was able to produce $2{\cdot}5 \times 10^{11}$ units (about 1 g) of interferon per year, using leukocytes from 90 000 blood donors (Cantell, 1979). This interferon, at a purity level of 0·5–1%, was the first and until recently the only interferon available for human trials, and Hans Strander had used it in the treatment of osteosarcoma, a type of bone cancer. It was, in fact, the overoptimistic interpretation of these early results that had led to the hope that interferon might be a potent anticancer drug, and encouraged the American Cancer Society and the National Cancer Institute to sponsor interferon trials in the USA (*The Wall Street Journal*, December 6, 1979). In this connection, the high price of interferon, purportedly between five and 50 million dollars per gram, became widely known, and likely encouraged the belief that the compound must be highly effective. I telephoned Kari Cantell, fully expecting to hear that he was already collaborating with one of the many potent cloning groups I knew to be interested in interferon. To my surprise he was not, and in fact I even gained the impression that he was not fully aware of the potential of the emerging recombinant DNA field. Worse yet, he did not know of me and was certainly not interested to come to Zürich to give a seminar, but yes, he would be interested to hear more about the cloning project. I flew over to see him the day after next, not only because of my hurry to get started but also to impress on him the urgency of our undertaking. This was the second advantage of my association with Biogen: I did not have to apply for funds or justify their use when a trip or some other unexpected expenditure seemed appropriate to me. Not that the University and the national granting agencies had not always been very generous to our lab—I was just reluctant to spend public funds carelessly, and I had a different feeling in regard to money provided by venture capitalists. If they wanted to risk their money I had no qualms about aiding them.

Kari Cantell became very interested in the project and pledged his full support, although I gained the impression that he did not believe that the undertaking would be successful—but then again, neither did I. We started out by determining the relative interferon mRNA levels of leukocytes at different times after induction and the sedimentation coefficient of the RNA. Peter Curtis flew to Helsinki for a day, with distilled phenol, recrystallized SDS and all other reagents required to extract the RNA from the leukocytes Kari prepared, and returned with the samples for further processing; the analysis of interferon levels was again carried out in Helsinki. We discovered an unexpected advantage of leukocytes: the level of poly (A) RNA was about one-tenth that of normal growing cells, presumably because the leukocytes, as nongrowing cells, did not synthesize much protein. Therefore, the interferon mRNA constituted a larger fraction of the poly (A) RNA than it would in growing cells, such as lymphoblastoid cells. On the basis of indirect calculations, such as estimating the number of interferon mRNA molecules from the amount of interferon produced in oocytes injected with a known amount of poly (A) RNA, and using the relationship found for globin as reference, we concluded that the interferon mRNA might constitute 10^{-3}–10^{-4} of the poly (A) RNA, and took the lower number as the basis for our further projections. In fact, the higher number ultimately proved to be the correct one. Peter Curtis spent a month or two trying to purify the interferon mRNA by polyacrylamide gel electrophoresis, and although substantial enrichment could be attained, the yields of biologically active RNA from the gels were very variable. I decided that we would carry out the cloning with the 12 S fraction of sucrose gradient purified poly (A) RNA, which was about ten-fold enriched in interferon mRNA, rather than spend much more time on purification. Peter Curtis, who had accepted a position at the Wistar Institute, left in October 1978 and Tada Taniguchi, one of the most gifted students to graduate from our department, who had up to then been pursuing the mouse interferon project, and Shigekazu Nagata, like Tada a veteran of site-directed mutagenesis in $Q\beta$ RNA, continued to work with the human mRNA. In addition, Lorraine Johnsrud, a former student of Wally Gilbert, who had done some elegant work on insertion sequences, joined us in September 1978. Unfortunately Tada was about to leave, and even more unfortunately he intended to continue cloning interferon in Japan, albeit fibroblast interferon. Since after Tada's departure none of my

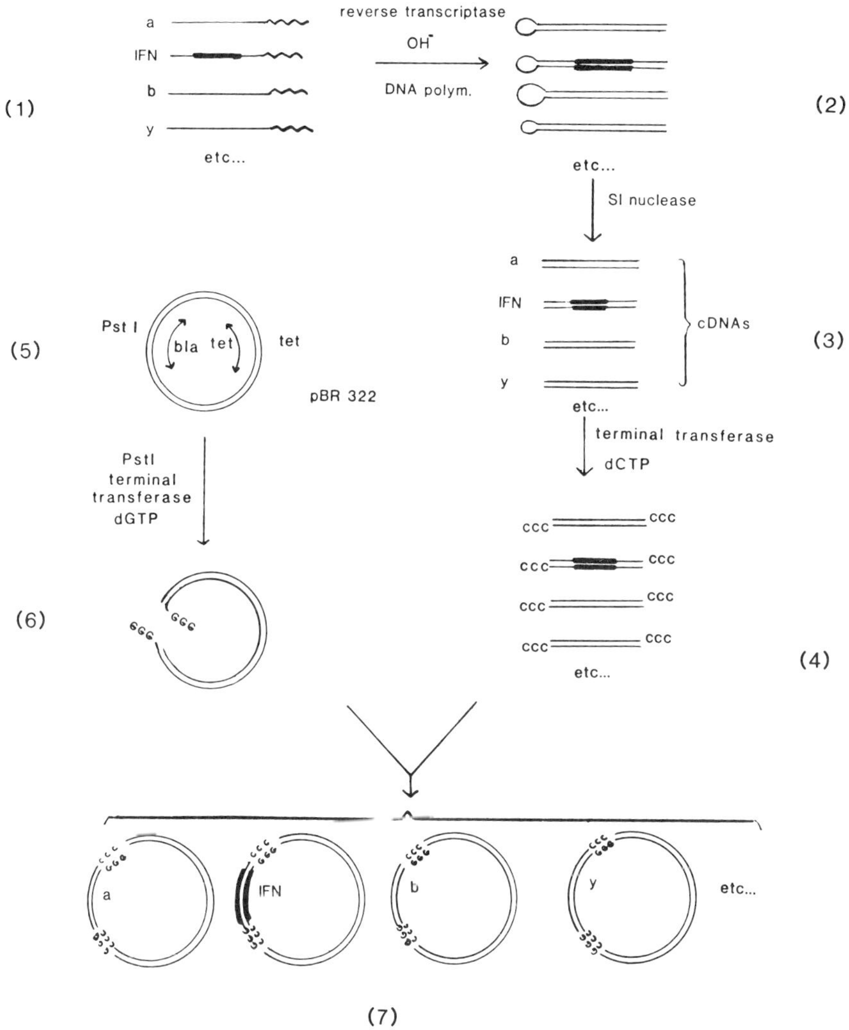

Fig. 1 Shot-gun cloning of cDNA sequences derived from leukocyte poly (A). Poly (A) RNA from Sendai virus-induced leukocytes (which contain a variety of mRNAs, a, b, . . . y, etc. and a small amount of IFN mRNA) was centrifuged through a sucrose gradient and the 12 S fraction (1) copied into single stranded cDNA using reverse transcriptase. After removal of the RNA by alkali treatment, this DNA was converted to double stranded DNA using DNA polymerase, which attaches to the 3′ end of the template and thereby generates a DNA loop (2). After cleavage with nuclease S_1, which is specific for single stranded DNA (3), the 3′ ends were elongated with dCMP residues, using terminal transferase and dCTP (4). Plasmid pBR322 (bla, β-lactamase gene; tet, tetracycline resistance gene) (5) was cleaved with endonuclease PstI, the 3′ ends were elongated with dGMP residues, using terminal transferase and dGTP (6), and hybridized with the dCMP-elongated cDNA. The hybrids (7) were introduced into *E. coli*, and 10 000 tetracycline resistant bacterial colonies were picked into the wells of microtitre plates.

colleagues had experience in making large scale RNA preparations, I went to Helsinki, and Kari and I spent a long night making leukocyte RNA from 10^{11} leukocytes, which I then purified in Zürich with Lorraine Johnsrud. Nagata prepared cDNA from the 12 S poly A RNA fraction, tailed it with dC residues, and joined it to the plasmid pBR322, which had been cleaved with PstI and elongated with dG residues (Fig. 1). This approach was chosen because the PstI site is located in the β-lactamase gene of pBR322 and insertion of cDNA into this position could give rise to interferon as a fused protein (cf. Villa-Komaroff *et al.*, 1978).

IV CASING THE BANK

Ten thousand clones of *E. coli* χ 1776, transformed with hybrid plasmids, were picked individually under P3 conditions (the Guidelines had meanwhile been relaxed) into microtitre plates by Nagata and Michel Streuli, an undergraduate student from Tufts University, who had joined us for a year to gain exposure to the vicissitudes of research. We pooled groups of 512 clones, Josef Ecsödi prepared the plasmid DNA from 12 such groups, and Nagata carried out the hybridization assay described in Fig. 2. The eluted RNA had to be treated with DNase (to remove DNA leaching from the filter), purified over oligo(dT) cellulose, and concentrated to a few microlitres, prior to injection into oocytes. This lengthy procedure entailed a substantial risk that the RNA might be damaged and for that reason give a negative result. We therefore added some rabbit β-globin cDNA to each filter, and rabbit globin mRNA to the leukocyte poly (A) RNA, and monitored the production of globin in the injected oocyte. This internal control revealed occasional failures of the assay and gave us a feeling for the background of unspecific binding to control filters. The assay was plagued both by occasional false negative and, worse yet, occasional false positive results. Nagata bravely toiled away injecting thousands of oocytes whose extracts were assayed in Helsinki. Time and again, one particular group of 512 clones gave a positive result, followed by several negative ones. Each experiment, from hybridization to the 'phone call from Finland, took about three weeks. We decided (and what choice did we have), that in the case of discrepancies we would consider a positive result as the correct answer, and a negative one as a failure of the assay. Thus, four of the groups of 512 clones (see Table I) were broken up into subgroups of 64 and the hybrid DNA analysed. While these analyses were going on we tried a short cut: Lorraine prepared bacterial extracts from about 100 pools of 64 bacterial clones each and Kari assayed them for interferon activity. Some pools gave a slight reduction of plaques in the assay but the results were not reproducible

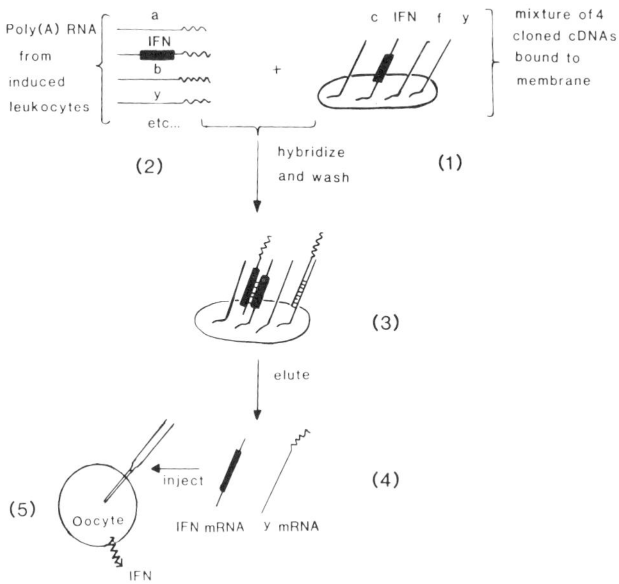

Fig. 2 An assay for hybrid plasmids containing interferon cDNA. Hybrid plasmid DNA from a pool of clones (see legend to Fig. 1) is linearized, denatured and attached to a nitrocellulose or a derivatized cellulose filter (Nagata *et al.*, 1980a). Poly (A) RNA from induced leukocytes (2) is hybridized to the filter-bound cDNA. If the mixture of cDNAs contains part or all of an interferon cDNA (or a sequence related to it), the interferon mRNA present in the poly (A) RNA will be retained on the filter (3) and can be eluted from it after denaturing the hybrids (4). Other mRNAs related to cDNA species bound to the filter will likewise be recovered, but do not disturb the assay. The poly (A) RNAs recovered from the filter are injected into *Xenopus* oocytes; if the sample contains interferon mRNA, the oocytes excrete interferon into the medium (5) (Colman and Morser, 1979).

and were impaired by a toxic effect of the extracts on the tissue culture cells. Since we did not really believe that this approach would be successful we dropped it after a few weeks. As we were to realize later, had the assay been more sensitive, or had we used smaller pools of clones, we would indeed have found an interferon-producing clone—a year earlier. We also undertook a further approach, in which we hybridized duplicate colony-carrying filters with cDNA probes made on poly (A) RNA from either induced or noninduced cells. Werner Boll, formally a technician but in reality a highly competent research scientist, spent considerable time on this approach, but the hybridization results were not reproducible and we could not decide which colonies were specifically hybridizing with "induced" cDNA.

The Biogen Scientific Board, which met every few months, patiently listened to my inconclusive reports, but other problems were arising which had to be dealt with urgently. For one, the co-founder and president of Biogen, Dan Adams, left the company at the beginning of 1979 following a disagreement with Inco, an important minority stockholder of Biogen, and the administration of Biogen remained in total disarray. For another, our financial resources were exhausted and at a certain point the company was technically bankrupt. Nonetheless, plans were being elaborated to set up a Biogen laboratory in Geneva and commitments were made in this direction. Luckily Wally Gilbert, who had been elected chairman of the Scientific Board, took over the duties of a chief executive officer and Moshe Alafi, one of the original venture capitalists backing Biogen, managed to interest Schering-Plough in our company. Thanks in large part to these efforts Biogen survived the crisis, and on June 28, 1979 Schering invested eight million dollars in the company, obtaining in return the rights to leukocyte and fibroblast interferon as well as an observer seat on the Board which allowed them to look over our scientific shoulder. The investment permitted us to create the Biogen laboratory in Geneva and intensify research in the universities.

Meanwhile rumours were abounding: in turn, Michel Revel, Lee Hood, Sydney Pestka, Genentech, Dupont or Derek Burke were said to have cloned interferon cDNA; as experience had taught me, I discounted all rumours and hoped for the best. Lorraine left in August 1979 and Table I records the arduous progress of Nagata on his own. The subgroups of I, δ and N were negative (although the groups themselves had been positive), but λ-III was repeatedly positive and was therefore subdivided into sub-subgroups of eight. To our surprise, three of these gave positive results. We realized only later that this high frequency of positive sub-subgroups was due to the fact that the frequency of interferon cDNA clones was ten times greater than we had estimated. Most likely each group contained at least one clone and several substantially more than one, but the assay was not sensitive enough to detect groups containing only one or two clones. Thus, to our good fortune, my overestimation of the sensitivity of the assay and underestimation of the interferon mRNA content of leukocyte poly (A) RNA cancelled out, allowing us to reach our goal despite my inadequate judgement.

In September Taniguchi wrote from Japan to say that he had identified a fibroblast IFN clone by differential hybridization and by the same hybridization–translation analysis we were using, but I was disinclined to believe it because I considered the vagaries of the assay too great to warrant a firm identification.

The eight clones of λ-III-4 (the first sub-subgroup to give a positive result) were examined singly. At about this time we switched from Millipore to DBM (dibenzyloxymethyl) paper as support for the DNA and this resulted in recovery of cleaner RNA and lower unspecific backgrounds. Clone

TABLE I mRNA Selection Hybridization Assay for the Detection of IFN cDNA in Hybrid DNA from Pools of Transformed *E. coli*

DNA sample	Interferon activity
Expt 1: Pools of 512 clones	
I	<60 (<60); *110* (<20); <110 (<110); <110 (<110); <35 (<35)
δ	*20* (<20)
N	*35* (<20); <110 (<110); *200* (<110)
λ	<60 (<60); *60* (<20); <110 (<110); <110 (<110)
8 other groups negative	
Expt 2: Pools of 64 clones from sample λ	
λ-I	<35 (<35); <35 (<35)
λ-II	*130* (<30); <45 (<45)
λ-III	*225* (<35); *35* (<30); *35* (<30); *600* (<30); <20 (<20)
λ-IV	*85* (<35); <25 (<25)
λ-V to -VIII negative	
Expt 3: Pools of 8 clones from sample λ-III	
λ-III-I	<20 (<20); <20 (60); *35* (<30)
λ-III-2	<35 (<35); <30 (<30); *150* (<20); *600* (<35); *110* (60)
λ-III-3	<25 (<25); <30 (<30)
λ-III-4	*30* (<30); <20 (<20); <20 (60)
λ-III-5 to -8 negative	
Expt 4: Single clones from sample λ-III-4	
λ-III-4-C	35 (60); *60* (<35); *111* (<11); <11 (<11); *20* (<20)

The number of bacterial clones indicated in the Table were transferred from the microtitre plates (see legend of Fig. 1) to agar plates, incubated for 24 h and washed off with medium. This suspension was used to inoculate 1-L cultures from which plasmid DNA was prepared. The hybridization-translation assay was carried out as described in the legend of Fig. 2. The values represent the interferon concentration (IU/ml) in the oocyte supernatants. The control values (in parentheses) were obtained with filters carrying only pBR322 DNA. Italicized values are considered positive. From Nagata *et al.* (1980a).

λ-III-4C was positive several times—but also negative on occasion. We used the cDNA insert of this clone as a radioactive probe and identified several cross-hybridizing clones in sub-subgroups λ-III-1, -2, -3 and -7, although some of these had never been positive in the hybridization–translation assay. I became very worried about these results—could it be that λ-III-4C had nothing to do with interferon cDNA and was binding interferon mRNA because it contained specially long dC or dG sequences, which might react with complementary sequences in the mRNA? Hapless Nagata (who was convinced he had the correct clone all along) had to carry out further control experiments in which he added oligo C to block these putative interactions—with no effect. Finally, Michel Streuli started doing the interferon determinations in our own lab by the cytopathic effect assay, and when I saw the protective effect of the oocyte supernatants with my own eyes I too became a believer in λ-III-4C—to an extent.

V A MERRY CHRISTMAS AND HAPPY NEW YEAR

Although hybrid DNA responding in the hybridization–translation assay fulfilled the criteria required of IFN-cDNA containing plasmids, the assay did not provide sufficient proof of identity because any cDNA fortuitously sharing some sequences with interferon mRNA, perhaps even in a non-coding region, could give a positive hybridization–translation assay. There were only two lines of proof I considered satisfactory. One was to determine the nucleotide sequence of the cloned DNA and compare the amino acid sequence derived from it with that of authentic leukocyte interferon. There was a rumour that Michael Hunkapiller and Lee Hood, using microgram quantities of lymphoblastoid interferon purified by Cathy Zoon and her colleagues (Zoon *et al.*, 1979), had determined the first 15 amino acids of the protein, however the sequence was not available to us at the time. The other proof would be to get expression of interferon in *E. coli* carrying the hybrid plasmid, a possibility I considered unlikely because I suspected that interferon, like other excreted proteins, would be synthesized as a preprotein in which the mature protein was preceded by a signal sequence, and thus might well be biologically inactive. In addition, leukocyte interferon was considered to be a glycoprotein, and we could not expect *E. coli* to glycosylate correctly a eukaryotic polypeptide. Therefore, if activity were contingent on correct glycosylation (although published data suggested the contrary: Bridgen *et al.*, 1977; Fujisawa *et al.*, 1978; Stewart *et al.*, 1979), the specific activity of interferon synthesized in *E. coli* might be too low for detection. Whatever we intended to do we needed a full-length cDNA, and since the cDNA in the original clone λ-III-4C was only about 320 nucleotides in length, we searched among cross-hybridizing clones for hybrids containing longer inserts. λ-III-2H had an insert of 900 nucleotides, which we thought might correspond to the full length interferon sequence. Hideharu Taira, a "postdoc" from Peter Lengyel's lab, the only person still working on the cloning of mouse interferon cDNA in our lab, abandoned his project and also joined the "human" group to characterize the λ-III-2H DNA by hybridization–translation. I talked Alan Hall, who had recently joined us, into preparing extracts of *E. coli* containing λ-III-2H DNA and other hybrid plasmids and test them for interferon activity. It was now around December 20, 1979, and after returning to the lab from our institutional Christmas party, Alan reported on the negative outcome of the assays. However, close inspection of the assay plate showed that some extracts had given a barely perceptible protection against the cytopathic effect of the virus. On further enquiry I learnt that the bacterial extracts had been substantially diluted prior to assaying, and since Alan had left for the Christmas vacations I now asked Michel Streuli to repeat the assay, however at a much higher concentration. Expecting a confirmation of the negative result, I departed on December 23 for a couple of days of skiing with my family. Next day I called Nagata from a phone booth on the top of the Alps and was thunderstruck by the news: a number of bacterial extracts had given strong antiviral protection at several dilutions! My comment, as Nagata recalls it, was simply "fantastic"! I rushed back to Zürich, stopping only to call Nagata a few times more to reassure myself of experimental details, and to call Moshe Alafi in Berkeley asking him to send over Biogen's patent attorney, Jim Haley, with whom I had already drafted the outline of a patent application several months earlier, based on the results accumulated up to that time.

Indeed, the assay plate (Fig. 3) was beautiful, and as I looked at it I experienced the feeling of utter bliss which comes only rarely in a scientific lifetime. I knew with certainty that we had achieved what I had hardly dared hope for, even though we still had to formally prove that the protective agent in the bacterial extracts was indeed an interferon-like substance. Since I had to leave for a meeting in Miami on January 4 and for the Biogen Scientific Board Meeting in Martinique on January 12, we were on a tight schedule. Nagata, Taira and I, the only ones left in the lab, characterized the interferon activity as being due to a trypsin-sensitive, acid-stable substance having almost the same elution profile on Sephadex as authentic leukocyte interferon. However, the critical test was the response of the bacterial activity to antibody directed against human leukocyte interferon. First I, then Taira (and two weeks later Kari Cantell) carried out the titration and to our delight found that the activity was neutralized by leukocyte interferon antibody we had obtained from Mogenson, through Kari Cantell, but not by fibroblast interferon antibody. While these experiments were going on, Jim Haley (who arrived on Christmas Day) and I were writing up the patent application and adding results to it as they came in. A secretary willing to type during the holidays had to be supplied with the handwritten pages in her home, and we were continuously rushing from the lab to the secretary and back at all hours. On January 3 all necessary experiments had been completed, and I left for Miami carrying with me the final draft of the patent application and polaroid slides of the results to show at the Biogen meeting. The final touches to the application were transmitted via long distance telephone calls between London and Miami, and Jim filed the documents on January 8, 1980. As all these developments had occurred during the Christmas vacations nobody outside the lab had learnt the news, except for Moshe Alafi and Jim Haley.

The meeting in Miami was on transformation of eukaryotic cells with

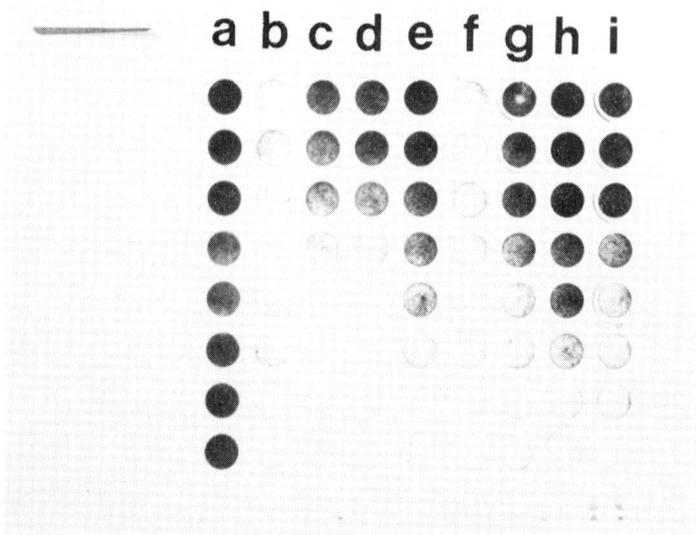

Fig. 3 Antiviral activity of crude extracts of bacteria containing interferon cDNA hybrid plasmids. Two hundred bacterial strains containing interferon cDNA hybrid plasmids were identified by a colony hybridization assay (Grunstein and Hogness, 1975) using the first interferon cDNA plasmid isolated (λ-III-4C) as radioactive probe. Bacterial cultures were centrifuged, the bacterial pellet was resuspended in a small volume, digested with lysozyme and the cells lysed by repeated freezing and thawing. The supernatants were assayed by the cytopathic effect reduction assay, using human cells challenged with Mengo virus. (a) control cells; (b) cells challenged with Mengo virus; (c) cells pretreated with 100 units/ml natural leukocyte interferon, serially diluted 1:3 or (d) to (i) with supernatants from the *E. coli* strains SN42, SN35, SN32, 287-2h-AH6, 280-2h-AH3 and 279-2h-AH8, serially diluted 1:3. (Assay carried out by Michel Streuli.)

cloned DNA, and I presented our work on expression of rabbit globin genes in mouse cells. I suppressed my urge to mention, just in passing, that we were planning to do similar experiments with the cloned human interferon gene, because the patent application had not yet been filed and because I was worried that if news of our achievement spread via the grapevine, our putative competitors might be stimulated to an all-out effort. From Miami I proceeded to the Biogen Scientific Board Meeting in Martinique where I presented to a largely unsuspecting audience the events of the last few weeks, which were acknowledged by appropriate expressions of glee. It was immediately proposed that a press conference be held to announce the expression of human interferon activity in *E. coli*, since this would be a unique opportunity for making Biogen known to the world in general (and to corporate investors in particular). In the ensuing discussion some of us expressed concern about an announcement preceding the publication of a paper, but we were all aware that if we waited until Genentech were successful we could be sure that they would not hesitate to inform the press and pre-empt Biogen. A compromise was reached: I would give a seminar at MIT and thereafter participate in a news conference. This approach seemed reasonable to me because the scientific aspects of our work would be subjected to critical scrutiny by my peers, prior to appearing in the lay press, not unlike what frequently occurs at a congress, where the speaker is interviewed by the press after an interesting presentation, following which the usual more or less inaccurate accounts appear.

VI INTERFERON HITS THE FAN

Since I had to leave for Zürich to start my lecture course at the latest by the night of January 16, i.e. in four days, a flurry of activities developed to organize my seminar and the news conference for January 16, no mean task in view of the difficulties inherent in placing a 'phone call from the Hotel to even the local airport. Transportation to Boston was another problem, and we were finally reduced to chartering a small four-seater plane to take us from Martinique to San Juan. I immediately bought a small typewriter (courtesy of Biogen) and started typing the manuscript for publication, since I wanted to be able to hand out copies to those colleagues or reporters interested in the more technical aspects. Typing in all spare moments, including the wait at the airport, I finished the paper during the trip back to Boston, on January 15. Next day, in the early afternoon, I gave my seminar at MIT, coyly entitled something like "Expression of eukaryotic genes in eukaryotic and prokaryotic cells". Despite the title the auditorium was overflowing, and I suspected that some news had preceded me. I spent half the talk on the globin gene transformation work and then, showing my improvised slides, I reported on the cloning and expression of interferon cDNA. Judging by the nature of the questions asked it was clear that the data had convinced the audience at MIT as it had convinced me, my collaborators and the Biogen Board. In the best of spirits I then proceeded to the Park Plaza Hotel to which a number of reporters had been enticed by a somewhat vague invitation promising news of great portent, issued by the Schering-Plough public relations department. I was accompanied by Wally Gilbert, who was going to participate in the presentation for reasons I was to appreciate only later, and Phil Sharp. In a somewhat dingy meeting room, overheated by lights and by a crowd of steaming reporters, Rob Cawthorn, chief executive officer and President of Biogen since several months, started the presentation by introducing Biogen and outlining its relationship to Inco and Schering-Plough. Wally then talked about Biogen's scientific plans and prior achievements, in particular the cloning of hepatitis virus DNA and the expression of hepatitis virus antigens by Ken Murray and his colleagues, and then introduced the subject of interferon, mentioning its scarcity and its potential therapeutic effect. In regard to the putative antitumour activity of interferon he said (and this is the complete quote):

> Secondly, at the moment there is a great, great interest in the use of interferon in the treatment of tumor; however again it is not known whether or not the leukocyte interferon is in fact truly a tumor active agent. There is enough encouragement in the current literature that there are wide spread clinical trials in this country of interferon as an anti-cancer agent. Those trials will take several years. There is no answer yet from them yet as to whether or not it is a truly effective agent, but the sort of the level of the problem posed by interferon, I can illustrate to you by pointing out to you that the American Cancer Society is spending some two million dollars on those trials and will only manage to treat some one hundred or so people. (Anon., 1980)

Wally's syntax may not have been great, but the description of the potential use of interferon was level-headed and accurate; nevertheless, we were subsequently often misquoted as having touted interferon as an anticancer agent in order to promote Biogen. Following Wally, I described the cloning and expression of interferon and then awaited what I expected to be an awe-struck response. However, one of the first questions was whether I had any reason for announcing our results to the press before publishing them in a scientific journal. A transcript of the press conference (Anon., 1980) records for posterity my suave response which started by "Yes, I think, I mean, I don't—" and continued in a similar vein to explain our motivation for the announcement. As the questions grew more hostile, Wally Gilbert gently unclenched my fist from the microphone and took firm control of the press conference. Eventually, all important aspects were dealt with accurately; we made it clear that the interferon produced in *E. coli* was most likely not chemically identical to natural interferon, in that it was somewhat larger (presumably because it had a signal sequence or was a fused protein), that it was produced at a level about a thousand times lower (about 20000 units per litre) than available from leukocytes cultures and—in response to a specific question—that we were convinced that we were the first to synthesize a compound with human interferon activity in *E. coli*, while others (and this referred to Tada albeit without naming him) had at most identified interferon cDNA-containing clones by hybridization procedures. With what turned out to be amazing insight, Wally predicted that within one to two years we would be able to manufacture interferon for clinical trials.

I left the press conference somewhat shaken and realized that had Wally, who was well known to the science writer community, not been present to put the full weight of his reputation and authority behind me, the claims of an unknown, seedily clad (despite a tie borrowed from a press agent) foreigner would not have carried much weight. Rob Cawthorn and I took the night plane and emerged bleary-eyed in Zürich to learn that the news had hit the fan with a vengeance, making the front page of most major newspapers in the USA, Japan, and Europe. In the first few days, fascination with the achievement (which was, to my annoyance, frequently attributed to "a Biogen scientist" or worse yet, to Wally Gilbert) predominated. The immense response was in fact not justified, however, the American press had been heavily primed for this forthcoming feature, the bacterial production of a priceless miracle drug; the stage had been set, largely by West Coast entrepreneurs, and when the curtain rose—albeit on the wrong cast—the success of the event was guaranteed. After some weeks, however, interest in the popular scientific features had worn off and a new aspect gained prominence in the newspapers—namely the news conference and my relationship to Biogen. I was surprised at the negative response to what in other fields had a long tradition in Switzerland and probably also elsewhere, namely the underwriting of university research to a significant extent by commercial companies and the issuing of patents to university scientists or the companies themselves. In any event, I experienced no discomfort as I had duly disclosed my commercial relationship with Biogen to the University before it was formalized, and a satisfactory agreement between Biogen and the University, covering the commercially oriented activities of my lab, has since been reached. The concerns of part of the scientific community were expressed in a scale ranging from thoughtful and balanced, as in an article of *Science* reporter Nicholas Wade (1980), to plaintive and ill-informed as in a threnody by Spyros Andreopoulous (1980) from the News Bureau of Stanford University, whose attempts to publicize Stanford's gene cloning achievements had fallen short of his aspirations, or emotional and vindictive, as in a pamphlet by a gifted microbial geneticist (but mediocre essayist) at the University of Geneva, which so far has failed to see the light of day but may doubtless be obtained in a plain brown wrapper from the author. Many of the problems raised in these articles are real and will have to be dealt with when the dust has settled and emotions have cooled.

VII LIFE AFTER CLONING

Upon returning to Zürich I submitted our paper to *Nature* where it appeared on March 27, 1980 (Nagata *et al.*, 1980a), the first report on the production of a human interferon-like protein in *E. coli*. In the meantime, preprints describing all essential features of the work, including detailed data on the restriction map of the interferon cDNA, had been sent to all scientists I knew to be working in the field (excepting only some commercial

S1 S10

1 10 20 30 40 50 60 70 80

met ala ser pro phe ala leu leu met val leu

G_{23}CTCTAGGTTCAGAGTCACCCATCTCAGCAAGCCCAGAAGTATCTGCAATATCTACGATGGCCTCGCCCTTTGCTTTACTGATGGTCCTG

HINF BSPI EcoRII AvaII •

S20 1 10

90 100 110 120 130 140 150 160 170

val val leu ser cys lys ser ser cys ser leu gly CYS ASP LEU PRO GLU THR HIS SER LEU ASP ASN ARG ARG THR LEU MET LEU LEU

GTGGTGCTCAGCTGCAAGTCAAGCTGCTCTCTGGGCTGTGATCTCCCTGAGACCCACAGCCTGGATAACAGGAGGACCTTGATGCTCCTG

DDEI PvuII AluI MBOI DDEI EcoPI EcoRII AvaII SFANI EcoRII
AluI

20 30 40

180 190 200 210 220 230 240 250 260

ALA GLN MET SER ARG ILE SER PRO SER SER CYS LEU MET ASP ARG HIS ASP PHE GLY PHE PRO GLN GLU GLU PHE ASP GLY ASN GLN PHE

GCACAAATGAGCAGAATCTCTCCTTCCTCCTGTCTGATGGACAGACATGACTTTGGATTTCCCCAGGAGGAGTTTGATGGCAACCAGTTC

HINF EcoRII

50 60 70

270 280 290 300 310 320 330 340 350

GLN LYS ALA PRO ALA ILE SER VAL LEU HIS GLU LEU ILE GLN GLN ILE PHE ASN LEU PHE THR THR LYS ASP SER SER ALA ALA TRP ASP

CAGAAGGCTCCAGCCATCTCTGTCCTCCATGAGCTGATCCAGCAGATCTTCAACCTCTTTACCACAAAAGATTCATCTGCTGCTTGGGAT

ALU MBOI / BGLII HINF
EcoP15 MBOI MBOII •

80 90 100

360 370 380 390 400 410 420 430 440

GLU ASP LEU LEU ASP LYS PHE CYS THR GLU LEU TYR GLN GLN LEU ASN ASP LEU GLU ALA CYS VAL MET GLN GLU GLU ARG VAL GLY GLU

GAGGACCTCCTAGACAAATTCTGCACCGAACTCTACCAGCAGCTGAATGACTTGGAAGCCTGTGTGATGCAGGAGGAGAGGGTGGGAGAA

AvaII EcoP15 PvuII SFANI
AluI

110 120 130

450 460 470 480 490 500 510 520 530

THR PRO LEU MET ASN ALA ASP SER ILE LEU ALA VAL LYS LYS TYR PHE ARG ARG ILE THR LEU TYR LEU THR GLU LYS LYS TYR SER PRO

ACTCCCCTGATGAATGCGGACTCCATCTTGGCTGTGAAGAAATACTTCCGAAGAATCACTCTCTATCTGACAGAGAAGAAATACAGCCCT

HINF MBOII MBOII MBOII
HINF

140 150 160 166

540 550 560 570 580 590 600 610 620

CYS ALA TRP GLU VAL VAL ARG ALA GLU ILE MET ARG SER LEU SER LEU SER THR ASN LEU GLN GLU ARG LEU ARG ARG LYS GLU

TGTGCCTGGGAGGTTGTCAGAGCAGAAATCATGAGATCCCTCTCTTTATCAACAAACTTGCAAGAAAGATTAAGGAGGAAGGAATAACAT

EcoRII MBOI

630 640 650 660 670 680 690 700 710

CTGGTCCAACATGAAAACAATTCTTATTGACTCATACACCAGGTCACGCTTTCATGAATTCTGTCATTTCAAAGACTCTCACCCCTGCTA

AvaII HINF EcoRII EcoRI HINF HPH

720 730 740 750 760 770 780 790 800

TAACTATGACCATGCTGATAAACTGATTTATCTATTTAAATATTTATTTAACTATTCATAAGATTTAAATTATTTTTGTTCATATAACGT

810 820 830 840 850 860 865

CATGTGCACCTTTACACTGTGGTTAGTGTAATAAAACATGTTCCTTATATTTACTCAAAAAAAC_{15}

AccI

competitors). Our lab was flooded with requests for interferon, often in the form of desperate letters, all of which I answered in an appropriate fashion. A seemingly endless stream of reporters requested interviews and information, and feeling guilty of having initiated the publicity, I felt obliged to clarify and explain the cloning of interferon to one and all. In the midst of this bedlam we intensively pushed ahead with the interferon project in four directions: elucidation of the structure of interferon, isolation of the chromosomal interferon gene, high level expression of a mature interferon, and fermentation and purification of interferon.

A The Structure of Interferon

Within weeks after isolating the interferon cDNA, its nucleotide sequence was determined and the amino acid sequence of leukocyte interferon was deduced (Fig. 4). A comparison with the sequence of the first 20 amino acids of natural interferon purified from lymphoblastoid cells, which had just been published by Zoon, Hood and their colleagues (Zoon *et al.*, 1980), showed that the first amino acid of natural interferon corresponded to the 24th codon of the cloned sequence, suggesting that interferon like so many other secreted proteins was synthesized as a preprotein, and that an amino terminal segment with 23 residues was cleaved off during maturation. We were disturbed by the finding that the sequences determined by Hood's and our group differed in five of 20 positions. A long 'phone conversation, during which I read off our sequence to Mike Hunkapiller and learnt some additional sequence data from him, led us to the conclusion that neither of us could have made that many errors and that there must exist at least two different genes for α interferon. Michel Streuli therefore started examining other interferon-producing bacterial clones in order to analyse additional interferon cDNAs. In the meantime, I had heard from Tada that he had almost finished the sequence of the cDNA he had isolated and that it encoded an amino acid sequence identical to that of β interferon from fibroblasts as far as the latter had been determined (Knight *et al.*, 1980). Thus, he could establish the identity of his cloned cDNA despite the failure to obtain expression of fibroblast interferon in *E. coli* up to that time. Tada and I agreed to publish the two sequences back to front in Gene (Mantei *et al.*, 1980; Taniguchi *et al.*, 1980), and Tada came to Zürich (on his way to Harvard, where he was to collaborate with Mark Ptashne on the expression

Fig. 4 The nucleotide sequence of interferon $\alpha 1$ cDNA. The nucleotide sequence of the insert of plasmid Hif-2H which contains the interferon $\alpha 1$ sequence, was determined by the method of Maxam and Gilbert (1977). The amino acid sequence was deduced from the nucleotide sequence; lower case letters indicate the putative signal polypeptide (S 1 to S 23). From Mantei *et al.* (1980).

of his clone) so that we could compare the two sequences. Sprawled on the carpet of my living room, we quickly found, to our delight, that α and β interferon were distinctly related, 29% of their residues being identical. We estimated that the two genes must have diverged some 500–1000 million years ago, and thus be as old as the vertebrates. The papers describing these results (Mantei *et al.*, 1980; Taniguchi *et al.*, 1980a,b) were also widely distributed as preprints, and several groups began attempts to synthesize interferon or parts of it chemically, albeit without succeeding in producing biologically active material to the time of writing; others again undertook to synthesize the gene chemically.

Michel Streuli found a cDNA clone with a restriction pattern distinctly different from that of the first one and when he determined its nucleotide sequence, the two were found to differ in 20% of their residues (Streuli *et al.*, 1980); again neither of them were identical with the partial sequence described by Zoon *et al.* (1980). It thus became clear that there had to exist at least three different genes for interferons of the leukocyte type. We realized that the multiple peaks of interferon activity described by Rubinstein *et al.* (1979) likely corresponded to products of different genes, and not to forms of one interferon differing merely in length and in degree of glycosylation, as was commonly thought. We were excited to find that interferon $\alpha 1$ and $\alpha 2$ differed in their host cell specificity, in that IFN-$\alpha 1$ was about ten times less active on human than on bovine cells, whereas IFN-$\alpha 2$ had about the same activity on both cell types (Stewart *et al.*, 1980; Streuli *et al.*, 1980). This suggested to us that the interferons might have different targets within one organism, but no other evidence in favour of this view has yet been reported. In any event it was clear that at least one of the species, interferon $\alpha 1$, had a number of the properties previously ascribed to the impure mixture of natural interferons, for example, activation of natural killer cells, inhibition of Daudi cell growth (Fig. 5), enhancement of antibody-dependent cell-mediated cytotoxicity, and suppression of antigen and mitogen-induced leukocyte migration inhibition (Masucci *et al.*, 1980).

B The Interferon Gene Family

Meanwhile I had obtained from Tom Maniatis his human gene bank, which had been prepared by partially cleaving the DNA of a single human embryo with HaeIII and AluI restriction nucleases and cloning the DNA in a phage lambda vector (Lawn *et al.*, 1978). As the human genome has about 3×10^9 base pairs and the average fragment size of the cloned DNA fragments was about 16 000 base pairs, it was expected that one phage in about 190 000 would contain an interferon gene, if there were one gene per haploid genome. By hybridizing 240 000 phage plaques with a labelled interferon

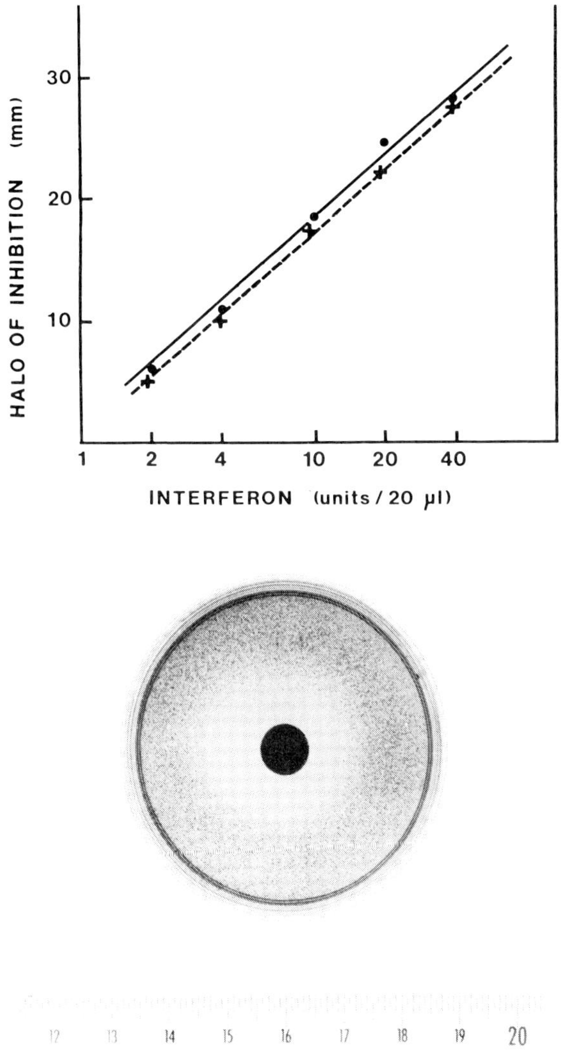

Fig. 5 Dose-response curve of growth inhibition of Daudi cells by interferon $\alpha 1$ (*E. coli*) and interferon from human leukocytes. Lymphoblastoid (Daudi) cells were seeded in agarose medium. Paper disks were soaked with 20 μl of the sample to be tested and placed on the cell overlay. After 10 days, the diameter of the halo, after subtraction of the diameter of the disk, was plotted as a function of the interferon concentration on the disk, expressed in international antiviral units per millimetre. Solid line, interferon $\alpha 1$ (*E. coli*); dashed line, control preparation of authentic leukocyte interferon (from K. Cantell) mixed with bacterial control extracts to give the same protein concentration as in the interferon $\alpha 1$ (*E. coli*) preparation. One unit of cell growth inhibition activity is the concentration giving an inhibition halo of 10 mm. The inset is a photograph of a halo of inhibition given by 10 international antiviral units of bacterial interferon. From Masucci *et al.* (1980).

cDNA probe (Fig. 6), Nagata identified 16 clones containing DNA related to interferon $\alpha 1$ cDNA, suggesting that there might be 10–15 interferon-related genes per haploid genome (Nagata *et al.*, 1980b). Restriction and sequence analyses of the cloned DNAs, as well as electron microscopic studies carried out by Christine Brack at the Basel Institute for Immunology in the course of the last year, led to the map shown in Fig. 7, in which 15

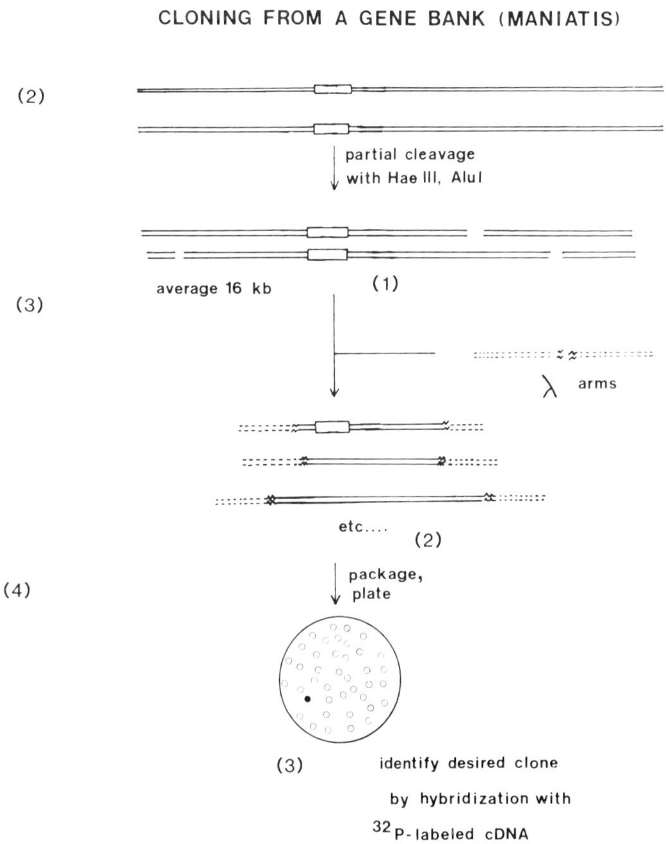

Fig. 6 Identification of cloned DNA fragments containing α interferon related genes in a human gene bank. Lawn *et al.* (1978) prepared chromosomal DNA from a single human embryo and cleaved it partially with endonuclease HaeIII and AluI to obtain an average fragment size of 16 kilobase pairs (1). The arms of phage λ were attached to the human DNA fragments (2) and the hybrid phage DNA packaged in preformed phage heads. The reconstituted hybrid phages were plated on a bacterial lawn, and phage plaques were blotted onto nitrocellulose membranes. Hybridization with ^{32}P-labelled IFN-$\alpha 1$ cDNA followed by autoradiography revealed plaques containing cloned chromosomal interferon $\alpha 1$ related DNA (3). The original plaque was then sought out using the autoradiogram as guide and the phage recloned several times.

different α interferon genes and pseudogenes are indicated (Brack *et al.*, in press). Altogether, as emerges from the sequence analyses carried out in our laboratories and by David Goeddel and his colleagues at Genentech (Fig. 8) (yes, Genentech eventually did get into the game, and with great vigour too), there exist at least 12 distinct interferon genes, which we consider to be nonallelic (Table II). In addition, several allelic variants of these genes were identified. Probably ten or more genes are expressed in man as judged by the fact that they give rise in *E. coli* to biologically active interferons and that in many cases the corresponding mRNAs occur in interferon-producing cells (Goeddel *et al.*, 1981). Allen and Fantes (1980) have, by amino acid sequence analysis, shown that interferon preparations from lymphoblastoid cells contain at least five different interferon species, of which one corresponds to $\alpha 2$, and another most likely to $\alpha 1$.

Beside the genes which have an intact coding sequence, a large number of so-called pseudogenes were identified, i.e. DNA sequences which are clearly related to functional genes but whose coding sequences contain mutations which prevent the expression of a full-length interferon-like protein. These mutations range from a single nucleotide substitution which introduces a premature termination signal into the coding region, to multiple, extensive insertions and deletions that mutilate the gene to virtual unrecognizability.

It seems that the gene family arose by duplication of an ancestral α interferon gene some 20–80 million years ago, and that further duplications occurred up to recent times; concurrently, genes were constantly degenerating as a consequence of deleterious mutations. The interferon gene family thus seems to be in a state of flux, with genes being created and destroyed over the millenia. We wonder if the maintenance of all these different genes has a purpose. Are different genes turned on in different tissues or in response to different stimuli? Do the gene products have different effects on one and the same cell type? Are they directed to different target cells or are we witnessing an evolutionary quirk, for which there is no selective advantage? All these questions can and will be answered; most likely there is a reason for the existence of multiple leukocyte interferons because the mouse, which probably diverged from the human line before the divergence of the leukocyte interferon genes, also possesses a family of such genes (N. Mantei, unpublished results), while the gene coding for fibroblast interferon $\beta 1$ is, at least in the human, a solitary gene (Tavernier *et al.*, 1981; Ohno and Taniguchi, 1981). I should note, however, that the data could also be explained differently, namely by assuming that the α gene family arose *before* human and mouse diverged, and that the genes of the α family were subsequently rendered more similar to each other by gene conversion.

A.

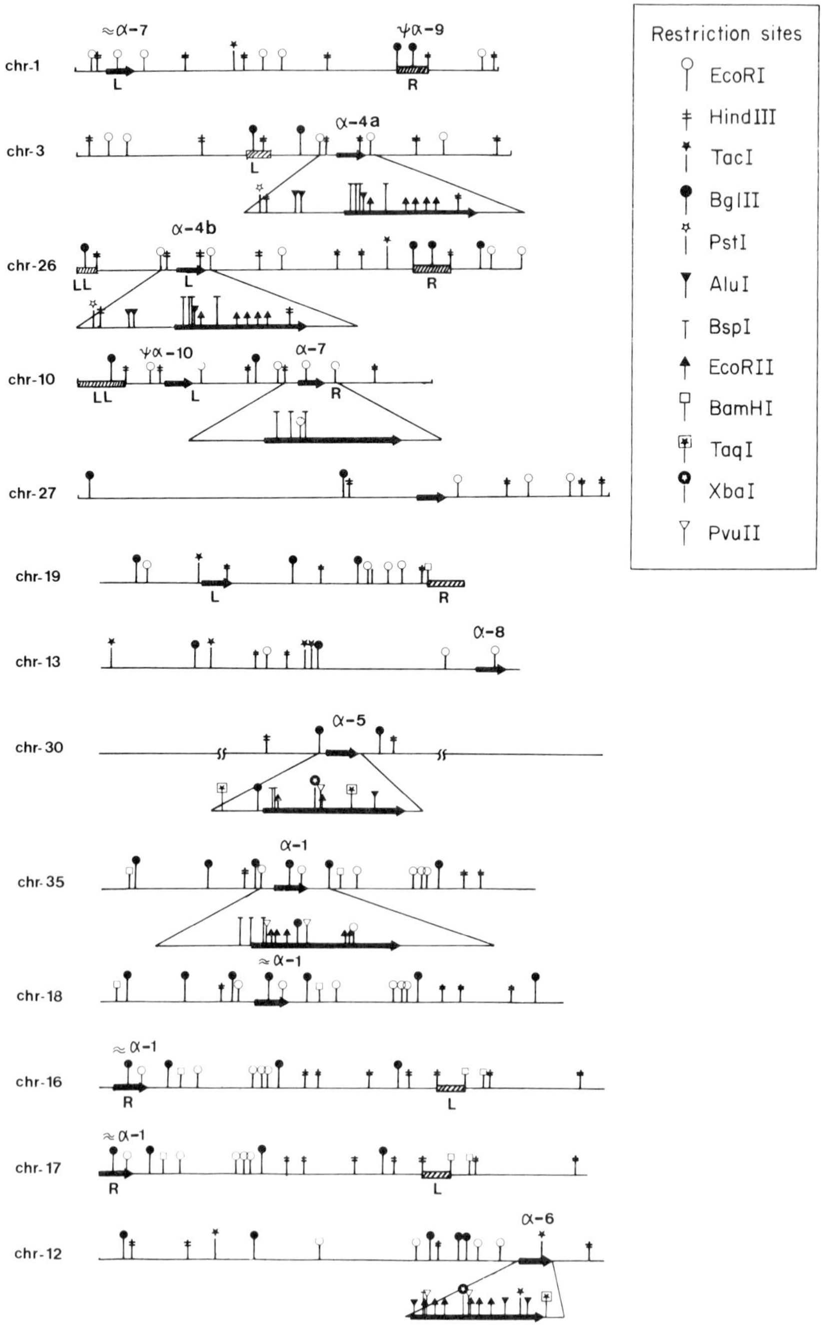

≈α-7
ψα-9
chr-1
L
R
α-4a
chr-3
L
α-4b
chr-26
LL
L
R
ψα-10
α-7
chr-10
LL
L
R
chr-27
chr-19
L
R
α-8
chr-13
α-5
chr-30
α-1
chr-35
≈α-1
chr-18
≈α-1
chr-16
R
L
≈α-1
chr-17
R
L
α-6
chr-12
Restriction sites
EcoRI
HindIII
TacI
BglII
PstI
AluI
BspI
EcoRII
BamHI
TaqI
XbaI
PvuII

B.

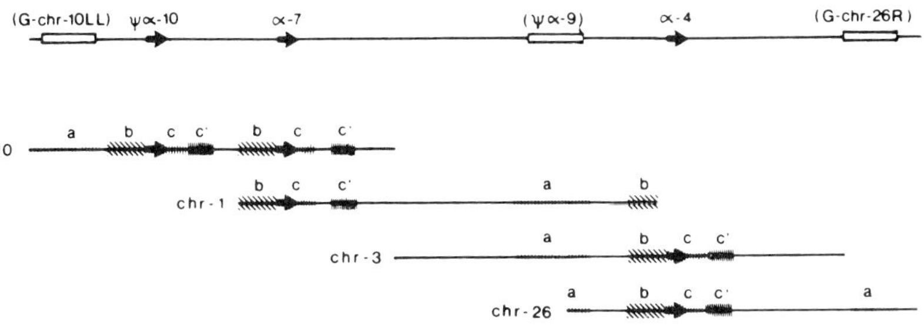

Fig. 7 Location of α interferon genes and pseudogenes on cloned fragments of human chromosomal DNA. A, the designation at the left of each line identifies the clone. Arrows indicate the orientation of the gene or pseudogene. Genes designated with α followed by a number have been sequenced; ψ indicates a pseudogene. = means that the gene is identical or very similar (allelic) to the gene with the same designation. Restriction sites are indicated by the key. B, from the data of (A) and heteroduplex mapping a partial linkage map could be constructed. The 36 kilobase pair DNA segment comprises 6 genes or pseudogenes: α4 and α6 are sequenced genes. ^{0}-α10 and ^{0}-α9 are sequenced pseudogenes. G-chr-10LL and G-chr-26R have not yet been sequenced. From Brack *et al.*, submitted.

A further surprise emerged from the sequence analysis of the interferon genes: none of them is interrupted by an intervening sequence (or intron) (Nagata *et al.*, 1980b), as are all other genes of higher eukaryotes with the sole exception (so far) of the histone genes. This brings a great advantage to the gene cloners, because it means that all chromosomal interferon genes can be directly expressed in *E. coli*, which is not the case for genes containing an intron in the coding sequence.

The greatest bonus of this work came quite recently, when Ned Mantei introduced the cloned human interferon α1 gene into mouse cells and showed that the integrated gene is under host cell control, i.e. it is expressed correctly only when the mouse cells are induced to produce their own interferon. This system will likely allow us to determine which part of the DNA is responsible for the control of interferon expression, one of the goals which initially enticed us into the field.

C Expression and Purification of Mature Interferon from *E. coli*

The strains of *E. coli* containing the interferon α1 cDNA in the PstI site of the plasmid pBR322 had relatively low levels of interferon activity, only a few molecules of the active protein per cell. The yield was rapidly increased about 1000-fold by inserting a DNA fragment containing the *lac* promoter at the beginning of the β galactosidase gene (Roberts *et al.*, 1979) in front of

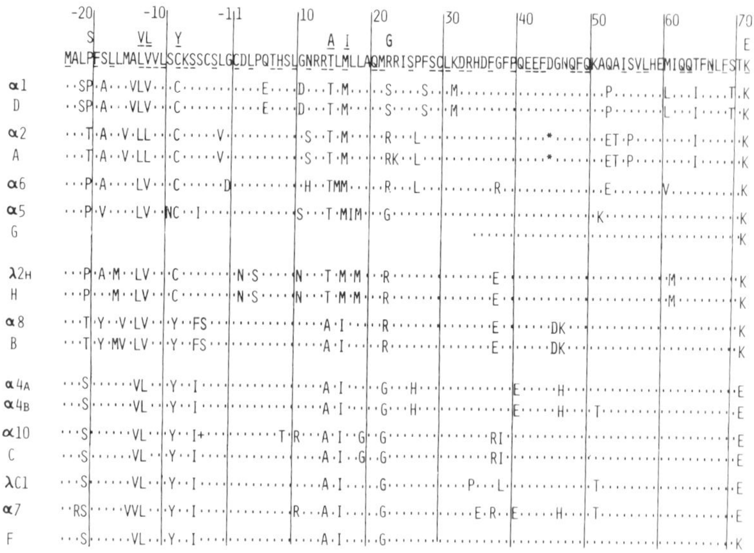

the interferon cDNA. The interferon polypeptide produced by this and similar constructions was preceded by part of the signal sequence and by a few amino acids of β galactosidase; in no case was the signal sequence cleaved off correctly in *E. coli*. Having anticipated this problem, we had already undertaken more elaborate constructions, in which the signal sequence of interferon $\alpha 2$ cDNA was removed and a *lac* or β lactamase promoter fused to the latter (M. Mishina, W. Boll and A. Hall, unpublished results) (see Fig. 9) such that the sequence coding for the mature protein was preceded by an AUG (initiator) triplet only. The resulting strains produced about 2×10^8 units (about 1 mg) of interferon per litre of culture. This interferon differed from authentic interferon only in that about half of the molecules carried a supernumerary amino terminal methionine residue. In October 1980 David Goeddel, Sidney Pestka and their colleagues (Goeddel *et al.*, 1980) reported that they too had cloned and expressed human leukocyte interferon in a similar fashion, and had obtained enough of it to inject three squirrel monkeys and demonstrate protection against viral infection. I was impressed (and stimulated) by the speed and efficiency with which the Genentech team had caught up with us in regard to the expression and preparation of interferon. Since Schering-Plough was not yet in a position to ferment *E. coli* on large scale, I undertook to work out a procedure for the fermentation and extraction of interferon which was compatible with the NIH Recombinant DNA Guidelines and could be applied on an industrial scale. The major problem we had to solve was how

```
              80        90        100       110       120       130       140       150       160
         EQS E  S                                                                   L F        D
DSSAAWDETLLDKFYTELYQQLNDLEACVIQEVGVEETPLMNEDSILAVRKYFQRITLYLTEKKYSPCAWEVVRAEIMRSFSLSTNLQKRLRRKE
α1   ......DED..D..C...........M..ER.G.....A.....K...R.......................L.L....E....E
D    ......DED..D..C...........M..ER.G.....V.....K...R.......................L.L....E....E
α2   ......DET..D..Y.............G...T....K.............K....................F.L....ES..S.E
A    ......DET..D..Y.............G...T....K.............K....................F.L....ES..S.E
α6   ...V..DER..D.LY...........M...W.GG..........................................F.S.R..E....E
α5   ....T.DET..D..Y..........MM.....D.....V....T.............................F.L.A..E....E
G    ....T.DET..D..Y..........MM.....D.....V....T.............................F.L.A..E....E
λ2H  N.....DET..E..YI..F..M...............K..........M.......................L.F...........D
H    N.....DET..E..YI..F..M.....................................M.................F.F...........D
α8   .....LDET..DE.YI..D.......S..M.....I.S...Y..................S...............F.L.I......KS.E
B    .....LDET..DE.YI..D.......VLCD.....I.S...Y..................S...............F.L.I......KS.E
α4A  ......EQS..E..S..............................................                          ...D
α4B  ......EQS..E..S........................V....................................L.F...........D
α10  ......EQS..E..S..I..............(-)...............I.R........................L.F...........D
C    ......EQS..E..S..................................I.R........................L.F...........D
λC1  ......EQS..E..S.......N..........M............................................L.F.....I....D
α7   ......EQS..E..S.....................F...........M.............................F.F....K.G....D
F    ....T.EQS..E..S...N.....M...........V.....K.....................................F.L.KIF.E....E
```

Fig. 8 Amino acid sequences of α interferons. All sequences have been derived from the nucleotide sequences of cloned cDNAs or chromosomal DNAs. Sequences designated with letters are from work by the Genentech group (Goeddel *et al.*, 1981; Lawn *et al.*, 1981); the sequences designated with arabic numerals were determined by Mantei *et al.* (1980) (IFN-α1), Streuli *et al.* (1980) (IFN-α2), A. Schamböck (IFN-α1), K. Henco (IFN-α4b), J. Fujisawa (IFN-(IFN-α5), J. Schmid (IFN-α6), T. Kovacic (Biogen SA, Geneva) (IFN-α7), M. Pasek (Biogen SA, Geneva) (IFN-α8), and J. Hochstadt and J. Brosius (Harvard University Biological Laboratories) (IFN-α10).

to kill the bacteria prior to removing them from the fermentor in such a way that interferon could still be extracted in an active form. Cathy Schein, Josef Ecsödi and I worked on this—once again man-made—problem for several months, and finally came up with an elegant solution which allowed us to scale up fermentation first to the 3000 litre level, in Brian Hartley's pilot plant at Imperial College, and then to the 30 000 litre level at an industrial fermentation plant which we rented for the occasion. With M. Fountoulakis we also worked out a purification procedure that could be comfortably used at this or an even greater scale, and yielded virtually pure interferon (Fig. 10a) which has been crystallized by Drs T. Unge and B. Strandberg (Uppsala) (Fig. 10b). Such preparations have been tested successfully in the rhesus monkey by Huub Schellekens and found to be completely nontoxic at many times the dosage required to fully prevent lesion formation following inoculation with vaccinia (Schellekens *et al.*, 1981), and have recently entered clinical trials. With this, the goals formulated with Biogen in 1978 (". . . to clone and express human

TABLE 2 Interferon Genes and Pseudogenes

(1) Genes closely related to IFN-α1		
(a) Sequenced and correlated with Genentech sequences		
Zürich		*Genentech Inc. (USA)*
IFN-α1	=	IFN-D
IFN-α2	=	IFN-A
IFN-α3[a]	≃	IFN-F
IFN-α5	=	IFN-G
IFN-α8	=	IFN-B
ψIFN-α10	≃	IFN-C
(b) Sequenced but not correlated		
IFN-α4		IFN-E
IFN-α6		IFN-H
IFN-α7		IFN-I
(c) Not sequenced but different from above		
G-chr-19		
G-chr-27		
Altogether at least 12 genes and pseudogenes		
(2) Genes distantly related to IFN-α1		
(a) Sequenced		
ψIFN-α9		
ψIFN-α11		
ψIFN-α12		
(b) Not sequenced		
G-chr-10		
G-chr-26R		
G-chr-19R		
G-chr-16		
Altogether at least 7 genes and pseudogenes		

[a] This designation was assigned to the protein sequence of Zoon *et al.* (1980). The gene has not been sequenced in Zürich.

leukocyte interferon, and develop a product accepted by the human organism . . .'') has been completed.

VIII WHAT NEXT?

As discussed above, interferon preparations derived from natural leukocytes or lymphoblastoid cells consist of about ten different species, present in unequal proportions, which are difficult to separate preparatively. The cloning of the genes and their expression in *E. coli* makes it possible to isolate each interferon species and examine its properties

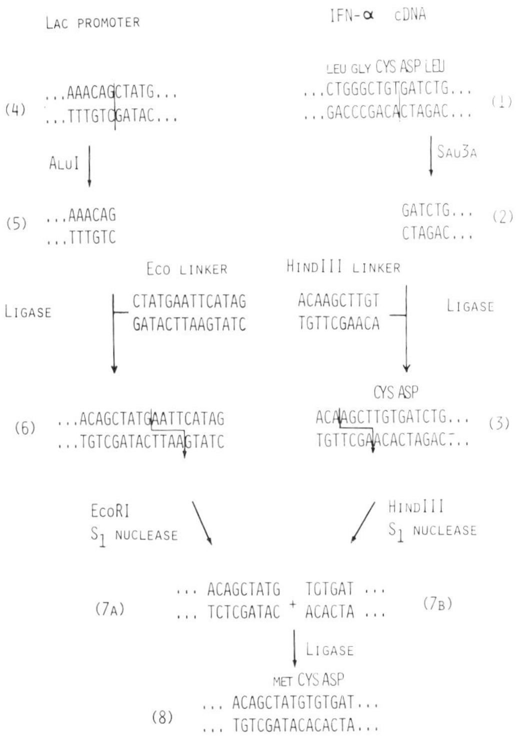

Fig. 9 Construction of a hybrid plasmid encoding methionyl-interferon $\alpha 2$. The coding sequence of interferon $\alpha 2$ (1) was cleaved at the Sau3a site (2) located between the codon for the first and second amino acid of the mature interferon sequence, and a synthetic oligonucleotide (HindIII linker) was ligated to the cleaved end, reconstructing the first (cysteine) codon and adding a HindIII cleavage site (3). A bacterial promoter-containing DNA fragment derived from the *lac* operon (4) was cleaved at an AluI site preceding the AUG initiator triplet by 2 nucleotides (5), and a synthetic oligonucleotide (EcoRI linker) was ligated to the cut end reconstructing the original sequence to the end of the AUG triplet and adding an EcoRI site (6). The interferon sequence (3) was digested with HindIII and the single-strand specific nuclease S_1 to generate a flush end immediately preceding the cysteine codon (7b). The promoter sequence (6) was digested with EcoRI and S1 nuclease to give a flush end immediately following the initiator AUG codon. The two ends (7a) and (7b) were joined with DNA ligase to yield a sequence encoding mature interferon preceded by a methionine. When expressed in *E. coli*, about half the interferon molecules lose the methionine residue by post-translational cleavage.

separately and in combination. One major task is to determine the therapeutic potential of the interferons. Not only must an effective and safe dosage be determined, but this must be done separately for viral and neoplastic diseases, and for the different interferon species, using appropriate patient control groups. There are basically two approaches to the problem, especially with regard to cancer: either one uses patients in

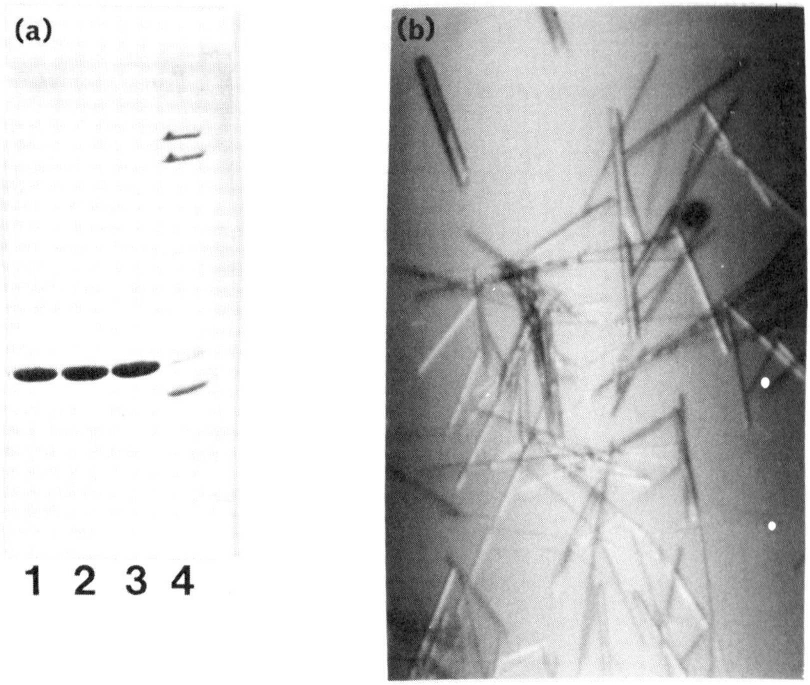

Fig. 10 Purified interferon α2 from *E. coli*. Interferon was purified from extracts of *E. coli* using chromatography on Matrex blue, Sephadex, phenylsepharose and DEAE columns. The specific activity of the preparation was 2 × 10^8 units/mg. (M. Fountoulakis, J. Ecsödi, C. Schein and C. Weissmann). (a) Sodium dodecylsulphate-polyacrylamide gel electrophoresis. Lanes 1–3, purified IFN-α2. Lane 4, molecular weight markers, from top to bottom: bovine serum albumin (68 000), catalase (60 000), β lactoglobulin (18 000), cytochrome C (13 000). (b) Photomicrograph of interferon α2 crystals prepared by T. Unge, S. Lövgren and B. Strandberg (The Wallenberg Laboratory, Uppsala).

an advanced stage of disease where other treatments are no longer effective, in which case a beneficial effect of interferon may be difficult to demonstrate because of high tumour load and diminished immunological defence, or one has to use interferon in combination with a conventional form of treatment, in which case large patient groups and long follow-ups will be required to discern the additional effect of interferon. Only if and when a distinct beneficial effect of interferon is found, can one substitute it for conventional treatment. If, as some suspect, only a fraction of all cancers were to respond to treatment, it might be possible to screen the response of tumour cells of individual patients in nude mice (Balkwill *et al.*, 1980) or even *in vitro* (Salmon *et al.*, 1978) and thus select patients for whom interferon treatment may be beneficial. Should interferon, at least in moderate doses, prove to be innocuous and to cause remissions of tumours

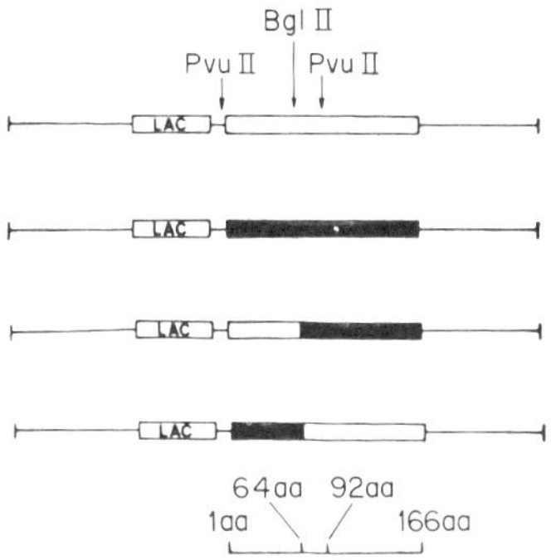

	IFN UNITS PER ML		
	HUMAN WISH	BOVINE MDBK	MOUSE L929
α-1	3500 (20)	17000 (100)	1800 (10)
α-2	25000 (190)	13000 (100)	60 (0.5)
α-1(B)α-2	100 (1.7)	6000 (100)	9 (0.15)
α-2(B)α-1	7000 (100)	7000 (100)	12000 (170)

Fig. 11 Target cell specificity of interferon α1, α2 and hybrids of interferons α1 and α2. Hybrid genes were prepared by joining the 5′ moiety of one gene with the 3′ moiety of another and vice versa. The interferons were expressed in *E. coli* under identical conditions and assayed on different target cells. From Streuli *et al.* (1981).

in a certain proportion of patients, it would be desirable to study the prophylactic effect of interferon, administered periodically for limited time spans, on a group of high risk cancer patients, for example heavy smokers or patients previously subjected to irradiation or chemotherapy.

We have shown that it is possible to construct hybrid genes and express the cognate hybrid interferons in *E. coli*. Figure 11 shows the structure of hybrids formed between interferon α1 and α2, and some of their biological properties. It is remarkable that some hybrid interferons have properties different from either parental molecule; for example, both interferon α1 and α2 have a lower activity on mouse cells than on human WISH or on bovine cells, but the hybrid molecule consisting of the amino terminal half of α2 and the carboxyterminal half of α1 has the highest activity on mouse cells. Using such reconstruction techniques as well as site-directed mutagenesis, it will perhaps be possible to tailor interferon with specific target specification or even selected functions, although it remains to be seen whether such unnatural compounds are antigenically inert in the human.

On the commercially oriented side, the cost-effectiveness of interferon production must still be optimized, which implies more productive strains (including microorganisms other than *E. coli*), cheaper media and more effective purification. As regards basic research, we still have to construct a complete map of the interferon gene family, a task which we are collaborating on with Dick Flavell. We have finally isolated a mouse IFN-α gene and are exploring the mouse system with Peter Lengyel. Much of our interest is devoted to identifying the sequences required for expression and control of expression of the interferon genes, using the techniques of reverse genetics (Weissmann, 1978; Weber *et al.*, 1981; Dierks *et al.*, 1981).

IX EPILOGUE

My decision to perform industrially oriented research in a University laboratory and to participate in the creation of Biogen was taken lightly, as I expected neither project to be successful. I have since asked myself whether I would have acted differently had I anticipated the outcome. On the negative side I count the adverse publicity and the critical attitude of many colleagues (although this consideration is mitigated by most of them having meanwhile also joined companies or started their own), the very heavy work load I ended up with, and the dilution of my interest in purely academic matters. On the other positive side, I had the satisfaction of applying my accumulated experience to create a potentially useful product, of learning industrial techniques and procedures I was hitherto wholly unfamiliar with, and helping create a company which may become commercially successful and—a most pleasant prospect—ultimately benefit me and my colleagues. Much of the recent work on strain improvement, fermentation and purification, could not have been carried out without the massive financial support by Biogen, since the costs were a multiple of our normal University research budget, and I would not have had the courage to request such sums from public agencies for a project whose ultimate outcome—both medical and commercial—was (and still is) so uncertain. Last but not least, the interferon project generated important spin-offs for the basic research in our laboratory, and financial support for the University. In going the way I did, I may have accelerated a controversial development which was taking place anyway, namely the involvement of academic scientists and University laboratories in industrial research. I have not drawn the bottom line on all of this, but it may well be that I would commit all my mistakes over again if given the choice.

X ACKNOWLEDGEMENTS

The research I have described came about thanks to the skill and enthusiasm of as gifted and loyal a group of collaborators as I have ever had the pleasure to work with. My special thanks go to the indefatigable Shige Nagata, Michel Streuli and Josef Ecsödi, and to our dedicated secretary, Rose-Marie von Rotz, whose organisational skill and resourcefulness time and again saved the day. I thank the Kanton of Zürich, the Schweizerische Nationalfonds and Biogen SA for financial support.

XI REFERENCES

Allen, G. and Fantes, K. H. (1980). *Nature, Lond.* **287**, 408–411.
Andreopoulous, J. (1980). *New Engl. J. Med.* **302**, 743–745.
Anon. (1980). Transcript of Press Conference, January 16, 1980, Boston. Roberts, Walsh & Company, Atkins-Kent Building, Suite 260, Northfield Avenue and Woods End West Orange, New Jersey 07052.
Balkwill, F., Taylor-Papadimitriou, J., Fantes, K. H. and Sebesteny, A. (1980). *Eur. J. Cancer* **16**, 569–573.
Brack, C., Nagata, S., Mantei, N. and Weissmann, C. *Gene*. In press.
Bridgen, P. J., Anfinsen, C. B., Corley, L., Bose, S., Zoon, K. C., Rüegg, U. T. and Buckler, C. E. (1977). *J. Biol. Chem.* **252**, 6585–6587.
Cantell, K. (1979). *In* "Interferon 1" (Ed. I. Gresser), pp. 1–28. Academic Press, London and New York.
Colman, A. and Morser, J. (1979). *Cell* **17**, 517–526.
Dierks, P., Wieringa, B., Marti, D., Reiser, J., van Ooyen, A., Meyer, F., Weber, H. and Weissmann, C. (1981). ICN-UCLA Symp. Developmental Genetics, Vol. 23, in Press.
Fujisawa, J., Iwakura, Y. and Kawade, Y. (1978). *J. Biol. Chem.* **253**, 8677–8679.
Goeddel, D. V., Yelverton, E., Ullrich, A., Heyneker, H. L., Miozzari, G., Holmes, W., Seeburg, P. H., Dull, T., May, L., Stebbing, N., Crea, R., Maeda, S., McCandliss, R., Sloma, A., Tabor, J. M., Gross, M., Familletti, P. C. and Pestka, S. (1980). *Nature, Lond.* **287**, 411–417.
Goeddel, D. V., Leung, D. W., Dull, T. J., Gross, M., Lawn, R. M., McCandliss, R., Seeburg, P. H., Ullrich, A., Yelverton, E. and Gray, P. W. (1981). *Nature, Lond.* **290**, 20–26.
Grunstein, M. and Hogness, D. S. (1975). *Proc. natn. Acad. Sci. U.S.A.* **72**, 3961–3965.
Harpold, M. M., Dobner, P. R., Evans, R. M. and Bancroft, F. C. (1978). *Nucl. Acids Res.* **5**, 2039–2053.
Knight, E. Jr, Hunkapiller, M. W., Korant, B. D., Hardy, R. W. F. and Hood, L. E. (1980). *Science, N.y.* **207**, 525–526.
Lawn, R. M., Fritsch, E. F., Parker, R. C., Blake, G. and Maniatis, T. (1978). *Cell* **15**, 1157–1174.
Lawn, R. M., Adelman, J., Dull, T. J., Gross, M., Goeddel, D. V. and Ullrich, A. (1981). *Science*, in press.
Mantei, N., Schwarzstein, M., Streuli, M., Panem, S., Nagata, S. and Weissmann, C. (1980). *Gene* **10**, 1–10.
Masucci, M. G., Szigeti, R., Klein, E., Klein, G., Gruest, J., Montagnier, L., Taira, H., Hall, A., Nagata, S. and Weissmann, C. (1980). *Science, N.Y.* **209**, 1431–1435.
Maxam, A. M. and Gilbert, W. (1977). *Proc. natn. Acad. Sci. U.S.A.* **74**, 560–564.
Nagata, S., Taira, H., Hall, A., Johnsrud, L., Streuli, M., Ecsödi, J., Boll, W., Cantell, K. and Weissmann, C. (1980a). *Nature, Lond.* **284**, 316–320.
Nagata, S., Mantei, N. and Weissmann, C. (1980b). *Nature, Lond.* **287**, 401–408.
Ohno, S. and Taniguchi, T. (1981). *Proc. natn. Acad. Sci. U.S.A.*, in press.
Reynolds, F. H. Jr, Premkumar, E. and Pitha, P. M. (1975). *Proc. natn. Acad. Sci. U.S.A.* **72**, 4881–4885.
Roberts, T. M., Kacich, R. and Ptashne, M. (1979). *Proc. natn. Acad. Sci. U.S.A.* **76**, 760–764.

Rubinstein, M., Rubinstein, S., Familletti, P. C., Müller, R. S., Waldman, A. A. and Pestka, S. (1979). *Proc. natn. Acad. Sci. U.S.A.* **76**, 640–644.

Salmon, S. E., Hamburger, A. W., Soehnlen, B., Durie, B. G. M., Alberts, D. S. and Moon, T. E. (1978). *New Engl. J. Med.* **298**, 1321–1327.

Schellekens, H., de Reus, A., Bolhuis, R., Fountoulakis, M., Schein, C., Ecsödi, J., Nagata, S. and Weissmann, C. (1981). *Nature, Lond.* **292**, 775–776.

Stewart II, W. E., Wiranowska-Stewart, M., Koistinen, V. and Cantell, K. (1979). *Virology* **97**, 473–476.

Stewart II, W. E., Sarkar, F. H., Taira, H., Hall, A., Nagata, S. and Weissmann, C. (1980). *Gene* **11**, 181–186.

Streuli, M., Nagata, S. and Weissmann, C. (1980). *Science, N. Y.* **209**, 1343–1347.

Streuli, M., Hall, A., Boll, W., Stewart II, W. E., Nagata, S. and Weissmann, C. (1981). *Proc. natn. Acad. Sci. U.S.A.* **78**, 2848–2852.

Taniguchi, T., Mantei, N., Schwarzstein, M., Nagata, S., Muramatsu, M. and Weissmann, C. (1980a). *Nature, Lond.* **285**, 547–549.

Taniguchi, T., Ohno, S., Fuji-Kuriyama, Y. and Muramatsu, M. (1980b). *Gene* **10**, 11–15.

Tavernier, J., Derynck, R. and Fiers, W. (1981). *Nucl. Acids Res.* **9**, 461–471.

Villa-Komaroff, L., Efstratiadis, A., Broome, S., Lomedico, P., Tizard, R., Naber, S. P., Chick, W. L. and Gilbert, W. (1978). *Proc. natn. Acad. Sci. U.S.A.* **75**, 3727–3731.

Wade, N. (1980). *Science, N.Y.* **207**, 507.

Weber, H., Dierks, P., Meyer, F. van Ooyen, A., Dobkin, C., Abrescia, P., Kappeler, M., Meyhack, B., Zeltner, A., Mullen, E. E. and Weissmann, C. (1981). ICN-UCLA Symp. Developmental Genetics, Vol. 23, in press.

Weissmann, C. (1978). TIBS *3*, N109–N111.

Zoon, K. C., Smith, M. E., Bridgen, P. J., zur Nedden, D. and Anfinsen, C. B. (1979). *Proc. natn. Acad. Sci. U.S.A.* **76**, 5601–5605.

Zoon, K. C., Smith, M. E., Bridgen, P. J., Anfinsen, C. B., Hunkapiller, M. W. and Hood, L. E. (1980). *Science, N.Y.* **207**, 527–528.

Present Appraisal of and Future Hopes for the Clinical Utilization of Human Interferons

THOMAS C. MERIGAN

Division of Infectious Diseases, Department of Medicine, Stanford University School of Medicine, Stanford, California, USA

I INTRODUCTION

In *Interferon 1979*, Cantell reviewed the uses which have been made of his leukocyte interferon, and in *Interferon 1980*, Finter and Fantes defined the case for the clinical use of lymphoblastoid interferon. Now, in *Interferon 1981*, I have the responsibility of summarizing what has been done in the past, and what should be done with interferons clinically in the early 1980s. I first reviewed the clinical potential of interferon in 1967 (Merigan, 1967) and have spent the past decade working on this question in my own clinical investigations. The major question dealt with in my first review was "Interferon's clinical potential—fact or fancy?" I hope the reader will agree with me that we are at least closer to answering this question today.

Not surprisingly, in the light of our present understanding I find the speculative aspects of this paper harder to present than the summarization. Difficulties arise with the prediction of interferon's future uses, despite the well documented broad array of its actions upon viruses, cancer cells and immune functions (Stewart, 1979). This is because the most important question a physician considers in using a therapy is whether or not he is using the most appropriate agent for a given patient's clinical situation.

Despite the overoptimistic views of interferon's potential that have been voiced in the public press, the critical question is how interferon compares to available therapy in those clinical settings in which it has been used. These now include half a dozen viral infections in man, and an equal number of human malignancies. The clinician needs not only evidence of biological activity in these settings, but pertinent data and appropriate conclusions obtained from controlled trials which allow direct comparisons between interferon therapy and other available therapies. Very few such trials have been reported to date because of the limited supply of human interferon. On the other hand, the list of other available agents for therapy of these diseases has been growing rapidly with the advances that have been made during the last decade in both the area of chemical antiviral agents and in the increasingly complex field of clinical oncology.

However, the ubiquitous nature of interferon has allowed biologists, chemists, immunologists and virologists to perform *in vitro* and animal model studies, which suggest its potential. As I see it, interferon has probably been examined at the basic level more thoroughly than any other compound introduced into clinical investigation. Now that recombinant DNA-produced interferon has become available for clinical investigation as well as the lymphoblastoid cell product, we should begin to see larger, more definitive human trials which, if appropriate, could be extended to widespread clinical field applications. This is because large scale production is possible from both these sources, and presumably with increasing utilization the price of the material will decrease.

However, all this is perhaps getting ahead of my assignment which is to tell you where this field is, and where it is going. This account, in keeping with the style of this series, will be a highly personal view. Furthermore it will undoubtedly be stronger in the infectious diseases than in the oncology area because of my background and training. Nevertheless for the past five years I have worked closely with oncologists and thus I hope to tell you something of what their real needs are in trying to place interferon among the available therapies within their armamentarium. In addition cancer contrasts sharply with the often self-limited and short-term nature of most infectious diseases; therefore, significant results in oncology are really only measured in five year survival rates rather than short-term tumour shrinkage. However, only anecdotal single case observations over a period of time will allow investigators to become sufficiently convinced of the activity of any substance to subject it to controlled trials, and compare it to a placebo or the best available therapy. Furthermore, the antineoplastic action of interferon in man has not been widely studied until the last few years. Therefore it should not be surprising to the reader that we must extrapolate the future of interferon in treating malignancies from a smaller data base than in treating infectious diseases.

II CLINICAL TRIALS IN WHICH INTERFERON'S POTENTIAL HAS BEEN EVALUATED

The initial discovery of interferon involved a demonstration of its action against viruses, and from that time on its action was known to have a broad spectrum compared to other antiviral agents. Several reviews (Borden, 1979; Dunnick and Galasso *et al.*, 1979, 1980; Pollard *et al.*, 1980; Scott and Tyrrell, 1980) of clinical trials are already available, and this summary will be selective rather than comprehensive in order to allow space for the speculation and interpretation which are a feature of this series.

Interferon was initially considered for application against those viral pathogens for which vaccines had not been developed, or where other methods of control seemed inadequate. For example, although large quantities were required early studies indicated that respiratory viruses could be inhibited in volunteers by local instillation of leukocyte interferon (Merigan *et al.*, 1973). Later studies (Greenberg *et al.*, 1978) indicated that large quantities were required because of the rapid clearance of the material away from the respiratory epithelial cells which was to be protected by the interferon. A recent Japanese study (Imanishi *et al.*, 1980) supports a Russian report (Soloviev, 1969) indicating that much lower dosages are effective in modifying naturally acquired infection in the field. It seems likely that this area will be further studied with the larger quantities of interferon now produced by recombinant DNA. However if, as I feel, it is likely that frequent administration of higher dosages are required, then new delivery systems must be developed to keep the interferon in contact with the cells to be protected. Furthermore, frequent instillation of drops in the nose is not a feasible approach for epidemic respiratory disease, which is in an asymptomatic stage when prophylaxis needs to be attempted. Hopefully, novel local delivery mechanisms will be developed for constant release of interferon in the areas where protection is desired.

Both vaccinial and herpes simplex keratitis appeared to improve with local instillation of interferon in early anecdotal trials (Jones *et al.*, 1962; Patterson *et al.*, 1963). Furthermore, several controlled trials have indicated that leukocyte and fibroblast interferons (Sundmacher *et al.*, 1978) produce beneficial results in acute herpes simplex keratitis. However, a number of chemotherapeutics appear useful and safe for this purpose and interferons do not appear to be better than other available agents. A recently controlled trial in Israel is of interest because fibroblast interferon appeared to improve adenovirus keratitis (Romano *et al.*, 1980); and no other therapy is available for this disease. Another virus which causes eye disease in man for which no therapy is available is coxsackie virus A24 which is sensitive to interferon *in vitro* (Stanton *et al.*, 1977).

Another major area of interest is the use of interferon in the prophylaxis or early therapy of systemic herpes virus disease in man. As infection with these viruses is more severe for the immunosuppressed patient, it is not surprising that they are targeted for early interferon use. For example, our group has examined the efficacy of human leukocyte interferon (IFN-α) in the treatment of herpes zoster in patients with cancer. We tested the material in four placebo controlled, randomized double-blind trials, involving 120 patients with cancer, which we reported in two papers (Merigan *et al.*, 1978a; 1981). Initiation of a week of treatment, early in the course of zoster, resulted in limitation of local spread on the skin as well as visceral complications and distal cutaneous spread (Merigan *et al.*, 1978a). These beneficial results occurred concomitantly with the development of a normal level of varicella zoster-directed, cell-mediated (Merigan *et al.*, 1981) and humoral (Merigan *et al.*, 1978a) immunity in the treated patients. A shortened two day course of therapy in our most recent trials (Merigan *et al.*, 1981) only influenced distal cutaneous spread. It did not modify progression in the primary dermatome where the virus inoculum was high and large numbers of lesions were present before starting therapy. On the other hand, both distal cutaneous spread and postherpetic neuralgia, which are probably sequelae of virus infection and inflammation in the ganglia, were improved with the short-term treatment course. After a preliminary trial which suggested some benefit in visceral complications of chickenpox in leukaemic children (Arvin *et al.*, 1978), a national multicenter trial is underway in the USA to evaluate both early treatment and late prophylaxis.

Studies have been reported employing moderate dose human leukocyte interferon therapy prophylactically in renal transplant patients in order to prevent herpes virus reactivation. Under placebo controlled, randomized double-blind conditions, in which objective parameters were followed, significant beneficial effects were observed on herpes simplex, cytomegalovirus (CMV), and Epstein-Barr virus (EBV) reactivation (Cheeseman *et al.*, 1979, 1980). However, reactivation was not completely prevented and it was interesting that other factors modified the extent of the antiviral action, e.g. antilymphocyte globulin antagonized interferon's beneficial effects. Furthermore, after the first six weeks of transplant, when interferon therapy was stopped, herpes virus reactivations occurred with normal frequency. Thus, the interferon effect was only manifest during the specific period when it was given.

In one recently reported trial (Pazin *et al.*, 1979) interferon produced an inhibition of herpes simplex reactivation in normal individuals. Patients undergoing trigeminal ganglia surgery for treatment of tic douloureux showed diminished frequency and severity of herpes labialis lesions in the interferon treated group compared to a group given a placebo. Not surprisingly, no effect of this short-term therapy was noted on subsequent recurrences of herpes labialis (Haverkos *et al.*, 1980). Attempts are currently underway to extend this approach to the early treatment of herpes genital disease.

CMV infections in the neonate have been treated with leukocyte interferon (Arvin *et al.*, 1976; Emödi, 1974; O'Reilly *et al.*, 1976). Virus shedding was diminished during interferon treatment, usually returning to previous levels when interferon therapy was terminated. Therefore, as in renal transplants, the extent of herpes virus suppression was dependent on the amount of interferon utilized, and the antagonistic action of ongoing immunosuppressive factors. Although in a single case of congenital rubella vasculitis appeared to be improved by interferon administration (Larsson *et al.*, 1976), when quantitative studies of virus excretion were undertaken in several infants, interferon effects upon this virus were observed to be minimal (Arvin *et al.*, 1981). Specifically, when virus excretion in the pharynx and urine were measured in infected newborns, interferon administration did not lead to virus eradication. Whether or not clinically important aspects of disease might be improved will only be shown in future work. It seems likely that a continuing immunodeficiency is important in the establishment and perpetuation of this chronic infection, and is significant in preventing any *in vivo* action of interferon.

Another virus infection in which human leukocyte interferon has had more beneficial effects is chronic hepatitis B infection. In short-term studies, using adequate quantities of leukocyte interferon, several investigators have observed an acute suppressive effect on Dane particle production (Greenberg *et al.*, 1976; Weimar *et al.*, 1978, 1980; Scullard *et al.*, 1978). On the other hand, for enduring eradicaton of Dane particles in female patients treatment must be continued for several months (Scullard *et al.*, 1978c). In males frequent long-term eradication has only been observed when interferon is used in conjunction with adenine arabinoside (Scullard, 1981c). Such combination therapy has led to disappearance of infectivity for primates from serum (Scullard *et al.*, 1981a), as well as improvement in liver function and liver biopsy appearance (Scullard *et al.*, 1981b). However, we have observed a higher incidence of neurological complications of adenine arabinoside therapy in combination with interferon than when adenine arabinoside is given alone (Sacks *et al.*, 1981). Fortunately with careful management this toxicity can be avoided, and combination therapy is currently under test in a large scale double-blind placebo controlled trial to determine whether these anecdotal observations can be reproduced.

A number of potentially effective agents against human DNA viruses have been under development in recent years. Therefore, if interferon is to be clinically important, it must take its place against a background of very specifically directed chemotherapeutics able to inhibit virus replication. Alternatively, the perspective for interferon in RNA virus infections is different in that no effective agents have been demonstrated in the decade following the introduction of amantadine and its derivatives. Therefore it seems important to determine whether interferon may be useful in acute RNA virus disease, particularly as it occurs in the central nervous system. For example, the observation that rabies virus infection in primates can be diminished if interferon therapy commences well into the incubation period (Hilfenhaus *et al.*, 1975) should be followed up in man. Two rabies patients have been treated with moderate doses of human leukocyte interferon in Paris together with good cardiopulmonary support (R. Gibert, P. Atanasiu and C. Chany, 1976, pers. comm.). Their survival time does not seem to have been significantly increased. On the other hand, it is important to pursue this approach in patients who are identified earlier in the course of their infection than the French cases were, and to use larger doses of interferon including material directly injected into the cerebrospinal fluid space.

Studies are underway in England with measles virus infections which can be lethal in immunosuppressed patients (Dunnick and Galasso, 1979). This is a setting in which interferon might be uniquely active and the results of such work will be of great interest. Other respiratory infections caused by RNA viruses, including influenza and picornavirus and respiratory syncytial virus pneumonias, might be available for therapeutically directed studies if rapid viral diagnosis methods could be developed and made available to investigators with large clinics. A single laboratory worker who was accidentally infected with Ebola virus was treated with interferon in conjunction with hyperimmune globulin (Emond *et al.*, 1977). Although this patient survived, it is impossible to know what role interferon played in his survival. However, this class of viruses, as well as arenaviruses and arboviruses, should be studied with properly controlled trials, utilizing human leukocyte interferon in large doses early in the course of symptomatic disease.

It appears that scrapie infection in mice does not respond to interferon (Gresser and Pattison, 1968). Therefore, it is not surprising that patients with Creutzfeldt-Jakob encephalopathy were not benefited by human leukocyte interferon (Kovanen *et al.*, 1980). It seems likely that in these infections, as well as subacute sclerosing panencephalitis, the virus replicative cycle is different than the more productive cytocidal viruses. Hence, they do not appear to be susceptible to interferon.

Finally, it seems important to evaluate interferon in other disease states associated with RNA viruses in which the exact role of the virus in causing disease is not yet defined. These include myocarditis or even juvenile diabetes mellitus cases which have been associated with coxsackie virus infections. As the pathogenetic role of viruses in these entities has not been clarified, much work needs to be done to determine what states might be most approprite for the use of an antiviral. As these complications are not common, epidemiological factors which predict the occurrence of such complications in an individual patient would be desirable aids to therapeutic intervention. The fact that the first attempts (Rand *et al.*, 1981) to modify early juvenile diabetes mellitus failed should not discourage other workers, who have better methods of identifying those patients who are undergoing viral replication in the pancreas. A final possible area of enteroviral disease discussed earlier which might be amenable to therapeutic intervention is the epidemic haemorrhagic conjunctivitis caused by enterovirus (Langford *et al.*, 1980).

It is interesting that another chronic viral infection that appears to be affected by administration of interferon is papovavirus initiated juvenile laryngeal papilloma. In anecdotal cases, the shrinkage of these tumours continues as long as the interferon is administered, and this therapy appears potentially life-saving in some children where respiratory failure is imminent (Dunnick and Galasso, 1980). A controlled trial is required to prove the efficacy of this approach. Intralesional injection of fibroblast interferon also produced small but significant effects on the growth of penile warts, another papovavirus produced disease (Scott and Csonka, 1979). Leukocyte interferon given locally appears to improve skin tumours associated with epidermodysplasia vermiformis (Blanchet-Bardon *et al.*, 1981).

Strander's studies on the use of interferon in the prevention of relapse of osteogenic sarcoma are clearly pioneering and undoubtedly will be extended in the future (Strander, 1977). However, they are not simultaneously prospectively controlled, and claims of their efficacy are not widely accepted. The major problem which could not be anticipated is a recent change in natural history of osteogenic sarcoma which has now been documented following present day standard therapy (Taylor *et al.*, 1978). This prevents valid comparison of present results to the data from an untreated prior study period such as Strander had planned. On the other hand, these early studies certainly taught us about the side effects, pharmacokinetics and safety of long-term interferon administration, as well as providing much hope that interferon could be used to successfully modify malignancy. However, the acute effects Strander and his associates observed in open trials with multiple myeloma have proved to be more convincing because objective parameters or tumours were acutely modified (Mellstedt *et al.*, 1979).

Our own studies (Merigan *et al.*, 1978a) in nodular, poorly differentiated lymphocytic lymphoma, in which shrinkage of tumour was seen, also demonstrated an acute effect of interferon on established malignancy. Yet all these studies were carried out only with crude interferon and did not necessarily produce the striking effects which can be obtained by conventional therapy. Gutterman and his associates (Gutterman *et al.*, 1980) have confirmed the useful effects of human leukocyte interferon in the latter two malignancies and have extended the interferon approach to breast cancer, another tumour which is responsive to a variety of other modalities of therapy. The failure of leukocyte interferon to affect non-oat-cell lung carcinoma (Krown *et al.*, 1980) may be related to the dosage and stage of disease selected. This contrasts with the improvements noted by ultrasound, X-ray and endoscopic monitoring of patients with bladder carcinoma treated in Denmark with human leukocyte interferon (Osther *et al.*, 1980). In preliminary trials (Hill *et al.*, 1981) a few patients with acute leukaemia were treated with short courses of very large doses of leukocyte interferon with some reduction in white cell counts.

The multicenter American Cancer Society trials have achieved their primary goal in that they have demonstrated an effect of human leukocyte interferon on myeloma, lymphoma, breast carcinoma and in certain cases on malignant melanoma. The major difficulty, of course, is that none of these trials has provided direct comparison in the same patient population of interferon with conventional therapy. On the other hand, this is logical at this early stage of evaluation of an antitumour agent because optimum dosage levels and scheduling have not been determined for interferon's use in any of these malignancies.

Other types of interferon which have undergone preliminary evaluation in cancer include fibroblast interferon (IFN-β). This agent has been employed intravenously by German investigators in several patients with nasopharyngeal carcinoma, one of whom had a striking regression under long-term therapy (Treuner *et al.*, 1980). It is of interest that this latter subject is the only treated patient who subsequently developed antibodies to the interferon. That became apparent on repeated injection of the fibroblast material (Vallbracht *et al.*, 1981).

British investigators have carried out a study to determine the maximum tolerated doses of relatively highly purified lymphoblastoid interferon and to define its side effects (Priestman, 1980). With lymphoblastoid interferon the side effects and tolerance resemble that of partially purified leukocyte interferon. At least two patients demonstrated some evidence of tumour regression, and further trials with this material are underway.

One type of recombinant DNA-produced α interferon is under evaluation in cancer patients, using intramuscular administration, in small preliminary trials conducted by us and Dr Jordan Gutterman's group. The pharmacokinetics as reflected in the blood levels are similar to what would be expected with leukocyte interferon, and the side effects are generally similar to those produced by leukocyte interferon. Thus the results suggest that glycosylation (which is not carried out in the prokaryotic system) is not important in the pharmacokinetics and toxicity of leukocyte interferon. The major question of whether there is improved efficacy with the recombinant DNA-produced material has yet to be answered. In fact, as precise comparisons remain to be undertaken, this investigator would be enthusiastic about continued evaluation of leukocyte interferon in carefully standardized patient trials to determine whether it might have special benefits compared to the mixtures of interferon seen in lymphoblastoid interferon or the single α or β species that are produced with recombinant DNA techniques in bacteria.

After anecdotal observations in a few patients (Fog, 1979) a collaborative randomized trial of leukocyte interferon therapy has been initiated by the United States Multiple Sclerosis Society to determine if it can prevent relapses in patients with multiple sclerosis. All of these patients being studied in the placebo controlled trial in the USA have manifested previous relapses, and are being carefully followed clinically and for certain immunological parameters. The rationale for this trial was provided by observations (Arnason and Antel, 1978; Huddlestone and Oldstone, 1979; Bach *et al.*, 1980) that patients with multiple sclerosis had deficiencies in T suppressor lymphocyte activity which involved interferon production defects both chronically and in the immediate predisease exacerbation period.

Another area in which no disease etiology is known, but where further preliminary observations suggest possible benefit of interferon, is Crohn's disease of the gastro-intestinal tract. It is not known whether the favourable responses in four of five patients who have been treated has anything to do with the normalization of abnormal immune responses or improvement in important host defences which are involved with the disease (Vantrappen *et al.*, 1980).

In the rheumatic disease area (Kajander *et al.*, 1979) there was some initial hope for interferon therapy, but this has now been dampened by careful pathogenesis studies during natural disease. In auto-immune diseases, circulating levels of type II interferon (IFN-γ) have been associated with disease exacerbations in patients (Hooks *et al.*, 1979) and in NZB mice both IFN-α and IFN-γ potentiated disease severity (Engelman *et al.*, 1981). Therefore much more knowledge of pathogenesis will be required before any empirical trials should begin on auto-immune and rheumatic diseases, despite the fact that disordered regulation of immunity seems to be an important part of their disease manifestations. For example, it is even possible that the administration of anti IFN-γ might be the most useful experimental approach utilizing the interferon system in the auto-immune area.

III UNSETTLED ISSUES IN CLINICAL APPLICATIONS OF INTERFERON

One critical unsolved basic issue is, "Which is the right type of interferon to use in a given disease?" As we review results in specific diseases and project for the future, it is appropriate to examine the rationale behind each investigator's selection of interferon (Table I). This issue is going to be a greater problem in the future than it has been in the past when investigators literally worked with any materials which were made available to them, and in those patients with which they had expertise. This is a major issue now that we have not just three (α, β and γ) classes of interferon but will soon be trying to evaluate studies done with up to 9 α, 2 β, and 1 γ types of interferon alone and in various combinations.

TABLE I Unsettled issues in interferon applications

Best type of interferon, dosage regimen and patient
1. Optimum type for a given disease (IFN-$\alpha_{1\text{-}8}$, IFN-$\beta_{1\text{-}2}$, IFN-γ or mixtures)?
2. Best dosage, scheduling and duration?
3. Optimum route of administration? Systemic versus local use?
4. Best patients for good response? Role of interferon deficiencies or pretreatment prognostic variables in selection.

The idea of matching interferons to the disease being treated comes to the fore most clearly in the application of interferons derived from recombinant DNA, especially since we have become aware of the multiple molecular forms of the interferon through their purification and the isolation of their multiple genes (Dunnick *et al.*, 1981). Obviously the simplest and most likely effective approach would be to discover the functions of the various types of interferon and to use those functions in guiding the most appropriate clinical utilization. There are already clues as to a "tissue specificity" underlying the antiproliferative actions of various interferons (Einhorn and Strander, 1977). There undoubtedly will be much work in the next decade to determine if individual interferon species act preferentially on certain cells, tissues or organs through their relative affinities for certain specific cell surface receptors or other means. Lacking this information we begin trials empirically and hope that the most appropriate matching of drugs to disease will occur. We hope that *in vitro* tests at least will allow the development of appropriate rationale on which to formulate the most attractive mixtures of purified clone products to take into clinical trials.

Another basic issue in understanding the potential for interferon relates to differences in the way it acts normally in modifying disease compared to how we use it in patients. Generally for treatment we are guided to systemic application to reach clinically not yet apparent sites of potential involvement. But interferon's physiological role appears mainly to be a local product of inflammatory or parenchymal cells in the area of disease. This means that as we project the therapeutic ratio we are limited by the fact that interferon, given systematically, can also effect or inhibit functions in cells such as the bone marrow, which it does not usually reach when it is produced normally in local sites. Yet, the clinician must push ahead with the systemic approach to reach important visceral disease sites unless new specific techniques and rationale are developed for more stringent control of drug distribution.

Another question which we are also asking is, "What is an optimum dose to use in disease modification?" If we can take lessons from the development of the corticosteroids, this is likely to differ according to the nature and stage of the disease and type of molecule utilized in therapy. Most of interferon's toxicities are dosage dependent, and several of its actions are biphasic in response to time and dosage (Sonnenfeld *et al.*, 1978; Dolei *et al.*, 1980). The issue of the timing of interferon's use is even more complicated when one considers the possibility that it might best be used in combination with other agents which are active as antivirals or against cancers. Given these difficulties, different investigators are going to have different views. Thus, as long as enough material is made available to enough investigators, optimal regimens should eventually be established.

A final area for which we do not have the necessary relevant information for planning trials involves patient selection from those populations in which the most beneficial effect might be observed. We have seen that factors such as sex, concurrent or prior steroid therapy, pathologic variety of liver disease and Dane particle levels influence the outcome of antiviral therapy of chronic hepatits B (Scullard *et al.*, 1981c). Other important pretreatment factors which influence the outcome of therapy with interferon will become apparent with studies in other settings. Another relevant question is whether there are any diseases associated with an interferon deficiency state in man. It is quite possible that successful utilization of leukocyte interferon in the early treatment of herpes zoster (Merigan *et al.*, 1978a) is related to the fact that zoster patients with malignancy have been previously demonstrated to have a delayed local interferon production when they progress to disseminated cutaneous disease (Stevens and

Merigan, 1972). However, it is also quite possible that complete lifelong interferon deficiencies might prove lethal if they were to occur in embryogenesis or during organ development or repair. Such difficulties therefore would be expected in patients if interferon proves to be a vital control for differentiation (Rossi *et al.*, 1977). However it is also quite possible that various diseases or the ageing process might partially impair the interferon system, leading to a greater potential for morbidity or severity of other viral or neoplastic diseases. If such relationships exist and could be defined, they might suggest the most useful settings in which to give interferon as therapy. For example, there is limited evidence that both the malignant and nonmalignant complications of EBV disease seem to be associated with a specific interferon deficiency in congenitally immunodeficient individuals (Virelizier *et al.*, 1978). Thus it is appropriate in the next few years to gather further information on the interferon response occurring in human disease by studies of pathogenesis *in vivo*. Such efforts may yield interesting clues to the potentially most efficacious clinical uses of interferon.

Now that I have raised questions about what type of interferon, dosage, scheduling, method of delivery or disease setting might best be employed for interferon treatment, let us go on to analyse what studies seem most desirable in the future.

IV FUTURE DIRECTIONS FOR INTERFERON TRIALS

Obviously, when one plans future trials (Table II), one has to take into account what has been done in the past, what are the most important questions that remain and what seems to be a logical series of steps to approach the latter. Despite understandable differences in approach of various investigators, there are certain fundamental elements of rationale which ought to be shared (Table III). For example, if one is undertaking use of interferon as an antiviral, it is reasonable to perform first pharmacokinetic tests to determine whether interferon could reach the involved site with the planned therapy regimen, and that the virus to be treated is susceptible *in vitro* to interferon's action at levels which will be obtained at these sites. Moreover, if useful antiviral effects are to be expected in terms of minimizing pathology, pathogenesis studies, if possible, should indicate that continued virus replication is going on which would lead to continued pathology at the time therapy was to be started. It is also useful to have quantifiable parameters of virus replication other than clinical disease to objectively assess the effect of therapy. Furthermore, the amount of interferon given should represent a significant increase beyond that produced endogenously in the infection.

Given interferon's relationship with the immune system, it is difficult to

TABLE II Future directions for clinical trials with interferon

Controlled trials required in:
Herpes zoster in normal and immunosuppressed patients
Herpes genitalis
Symptomatic CMV and EBV infections
Rabies and other RNA viral CNS infections
Influenza, rhinoviral, respiratory syncytial or other respiratory viral infections
Adenovirus and picornoviral keratitis
Chronic hepatitis B virus infection
Tracheobronchial and cutaneous papovaviral infections
Phase 3 Controlled Trials
After phase 2 trials indicating efficacy in:
Acute cytoreductive therapy of various haematopoietic and solid tumours (in combination with or compared to standard therapy)
Long-term therapy to prevent relapse in high risk patients (e.g. patients successfully treated with other approaches or with early indications of tumour presence)

TABLE III Pharmacologic requirements for interferon studies

1. Pathogenetic data indicating continued viral replication at time treatment is started
2. Evidence that interferon can reach sites of replication at levels active against the agent *in vitro*
3. Availability of quantitative parameters to assess inhibition of viral replication
4. Amount of interferon given should be significantly greater than that present endogenously at the start of therapy

know whether beneficial results in malignancy relate to interferon's direct antiproliferative action on tumour cells or to heightened host defences. This issues is an important area for further investigation, and as many tumours should be grown *in vitro* as possible and tested with interferon, especially where the agent is concomitantly tested in the same patient. This may allow us to determine whether the *in vitro* sensitivity of a tumour cell might predict *in vivo* efficacy as is the case with certain chemotherapeutics (Salmon *et al.*, 1978).

A number of studies (Desmyter *et al.*, 1976; Weimar *et al.*, 1977, 1978; Billiau *et al.*, 1979b) were done with fibroblast interferon before pharmacokinetics were analysed. In retrospect, the pharmacokinetics (Billiau *et al.*, 1979a) indicated that it was very unlikely viral inhibitory doses reached the involved sites when intramuscular administration was utilized. Intramuscular treatment was initially undertaken in a manner similar to that found useful with leukocyte interferon. However, with the latter, early verification of lack of tissue binding and good uptake into the blood stream from the initial injection site was obtained before clinical investigations were carried out (Jordan *et al.*, 1974). To avoid misleading findings, it is strongly recommended that all new interferons be subjected to careful pharmacokinetic studies before attempting clinical utilization in disease.

In regard to acute infections, it is important to determine whether the observation of diminished postherpetic neuralgia in interferon treated cancer patients (Merigan *et al.*, 1978a) be extended to normal individuals. Postherpetic neuralgia is an important sequel to zoster, especially in the aged, and no other modality has been evaluated which reduced this effect, although it is possible that new agents under development, such as adenine arabinoside monophosphate or acycloguanosine, might have this potential.

In addition, as mentioned earlier, studies are still underway to determine if leukocyte interferon will modify the severity of primary or secondary herpes genital infections.

Therapies for other herpes viruses need further evaluation. These include attempts to treat symptomatic EBV infection in both certain normal individuals and in patients with X-linked lymphoproliferative disorders in whom the disease is often severe or prolonged (Sullivan *et al.*, 1980). CMV mononucleosis in certain normal individuals also represents an important clinical problem. The difficulty with these two viral infections is that they are of low frequency in a severe form and only cooperative multicenter trials would allow the proper controlled testing necessary to determine whether an acute effect on the disease could be observed.

As we have gained a good deal of knowledge on the effect of interferon in chronic hepatitis B infection, there is need to cautiously extend such studies into acute hepatitis B infection. It is possible that the frequency of chronic disease as well as acute pathology may be decreased if the disease is treated acutely. It would be important to evaluate at least 2–4 weeks of interferon therapy under a randomized controlled double-blind format to answer this question.

Randomized double-blind controlled trials should be carried out in adenovirus keratitis. It is also important to determine whether interferon can benefit central nervous system RNA viral infections, including rabies, as well as those due to arboviruses, arenaviruses and other exotic agents. After sufficient open trial experience is obtained, it is recommended that controlled trials also be initiated in these areas.

In regard to chronic virus infections, because the dosing regimens are likely to be much longer and there are a greater number of variations involving drug pulsing and long-term versus low-dose therapy, study designs are more complex as in the treatment of malignancy. Chronic hepatitis B short-term treatment trials, which are placebo controlled, have already been reported (Weimar *et al.*, 1980). However, it is important not to carry out controlled trials until one has evidence of the most effective regimens from open study experience. Such investigations suggest that interferon may need to be combined with other agents in order to have optimum effects, and optimum treatment for hepatitis B may need to be as long as 6–12 months (Scullard *et al.*, 1981c). With such long-term trials, it seems to me that only after some years of investigation can one begin a large-scale controlled trial to evaluate efficacy. We are now beginning such a large-scale, long-term trial, involving adenine arabinoside monophosphate in combination with leukocyte interferon compared to adenine arabinoside monophosphate alone and to a placebo. We have included stratification within this three-limbed trial for a number of pretreatment variables which were found to influence the outcome of therapy in our open trials (Scullard *et al.*, 1981c).

The good response to leukocyte interferon of juvenile laryngeal papilloma in open trials (Dunnick and Galasso, 1980) suggests that a multicenter, randomized double-blind trial using a moderate dose against a placebo should be undertaken currently. On the other hand, in regard to two other chronic infections, CMV and HSV, our knowledge of various therapeutic approaches is not presently adequate. Before controlled trial attempts at virus eradication, further open trials are required. Interferon administration in CMV infection has been only associated with transient suppression of viuria. On the other hand, as other chemicals (Pollard *et al.*, 1980) are appearing which also act against this infection in immunosuppressed and newborn individuals, combination therapy needs to be undertaken as well as studies with new types of interferon made available through cloning technology. Only relatively rarely in cases of chronic herpes simplex disease is there a need for evaluation of long-term suppressive therapy both in terms of prevention of symptomatic recrudescent disease episodes as well as possible eradication of infection.

In the future, studies of interferon actions on cancer will undoubtedly be carried on in a number of malignancies. Trials in which interferon is combined with or compared to other conventional therapies should be undertaken under carefully controlled conditions. As with chronic hepatitis, some time may have to elapse before those definitive trials get underway. We hope that additional knowledge from *in vitro* pharmacokinetic or immunological monitoring studies in man will provide important rationales for the selection of regimens chosen for such controlled trials.

It seems especially important to follow up in man the evidence that interferon therapy produces at least additive and perhaps synergistic effects with cytocidal chemotherapy in inhibiting the development of leukaemias in mice (Chirigos and Pearson, 1973; Gresser *et al.*, 1976).

Another major area in malignancy control, where interferon seems likely to have a useful role, is in the prevention of malignancy in certain high risk individuals. This approach seems particularly physiological in that long-term administration of interferon may be possible because of its role in man as a natural defence mechanism. If one has markers for the early detection of malignancy, one could use low dosage interferon in a presymptomatic phase to try to control inapparent disease. Then one might be using the material in the most physiological and nontoxic manner, both at a time the tumour load is low and when host defences are most likely to be intact. Data have been produced in the People's Republic of China that rising α fetoprotein levels in patients with chronic hepatitis B (Merigan, 1980) and elevated IgA antibody levels to EBV (Zeng *et al.*, 1979) predict the subsequent appearance of clinically detectable hepatocellular carcinoma and nasopharyngeal carcinoma respectively. Once interferon dosages which are active *in vivo* in such malignancies are determined, it seems worthwhile to try such regimens on a long-term randomized controlled basis against a placebo in the high risk individuals to see if one can prevent the occurrence of clinically apparent disease. Long-term administration of interferon to maintain remissions produced by other modalities also must be tested in controlled trials in patients with a variety of interferon sensitive malignant diseases.

As one reviews all these possibilities, it is apparent that there is much more work that can be accomplished in our lifetime. Undoubtedly, all of our enthusiasm for such work will depend on the results of clinical trials which will be undertaken in the next few years. The efforts which we undertake hopefully will be benefited substantially by future basic science contributions yet to be made. Clearly, basic science, through recombinant DNA and large scale tissue culture methods, has made a major impact on the interferon area by solving the supply problem which was limiting previous clinical investigations.

V SUMMARY

This review has attempted to present the problems and the perspective for clinical applications of interferon. Encouraging results have been achieved in acute and chronic viral diseases with interferon and in various malignancies. Eukaryotic cell culture methodology on a large scale and recombinant DNA expression in bacterial systems have proved useful to suppliers of interferon for clinical trials. An unresolved issue is whether such efforts will have a practical outcome resulting in interferon becoming the agent of choice for at least a few human diseases. Given the breadth of its effects, it seems impossible that interferon will not find some place in human medicine. But on the other hand, much work needs to be done to clarify exactly what its clinical applications will be in the future.

VI ACKNOWLEDGEMENTS

Supported by a grant (AI-05629) and contracts (AI-42527, NCI-CM-07343-22) from the United States Public Health Service and a grant from the Multiple Sclerosis Society (RG1287-A-1).

VII REFERENCES

Arnason, B. G. W. and Antel, J. (1978). *Ann. Immunol.* **129C**, 159–170.
Arvin, A. M., Yeager, A. S. and Merigan, T. C. (1976). *J. infect. Dis.* **133**, Suppl., A205–A210.
Arvin, A. M., Feldman, S. and Merigan, T. C. (1978). *Antimicrob. Agents Chemother.* **13**, 605–607.
Arvin, A. M., Schmidt, N., Cantell, K. and Merigan, T. C. (1981). In preparation.
Bach, M. A., Phan-Dinh-Tuy, F., Tournier, E., Chatenoud, L. and Bach, J. F. (1980). *Lancet* **ii**, 1221–1223.
Billiau, A., De Somer, P., Edy, V. G., DeClercq, E. and Heremans, H. (1979a). *Antimicrob. Agents Chemother.* **16**, 56–63.
Billiau, A., Edy, V. G. and Somer, P. (1979b). *In* "Antiviral Mechanisms in the Control of Neoplasia" pp. 675–696. Plenum Publishing, New York and London.
Blanchet-Bardon, C., Pruissant, A., Lutzner, M., Orth, G., Nutini, M. T. and Guesry, P. (1981). *Lancet* **i**, 274.
Borden, E. C. (1979). *Ann. intern. Med.* **91**, 472–479.
Cheeseman, S. H., Rubin, R. H., Stewart, J. A., Tolkoff, N. E., Cosimi, A. B., Cantell, K., Gilbert, J., Winkle, S., Herrin, J. T., Black, P. H., Russell, P. S. and Hirsch, M. D. (1979). *New Engl. J. Med.* **300**, 1345–1349.
Cheeseman, S. H., Henle, W., Rubin, R. H., Tolkoff-Rubin, N. E., Cosimi, G., Cantell, K., Winkle, S., Herrin, J. T., Black, P. H., Russell, P. S. and Hirsch, M. S. (1980). *Ann. intern. Med.* **93**, 39–42.
Chirigos, M. A. and Pearson, J. W. (1973). *J. natn. Cancer Inst.* **51**, 1367–1368.
Desmyter, J., De Groote, J. and Desmet, V. J. *et al.* (1976). *Lancet* **ii**, 645–647.
De Somer, P., Edy, V. G. and Billiau, A. (1977). *Lancet* **ii**, 47–48.
Dolei, A., Colleta, G., Copobianchi, M. R., Rossi, G. G. and Vecchio, G. (1980). *J. gen. Virol.* **46**, 227.
Dunnick, J. K. and Galasso, G. J. (1979). *J. infect. Dis.* **139**, 109–123.
Dunnick, J. K. and Galasso, G. J. (1980). *J. infect. Dis.* **142**, 293–299.
Dunnick, J. K., Merigan, T. C. and Galasso, G. J. (1981). *J. infect. Dis.* in press.
Einhorn, S. and Strander, H. (1977). *J. gen. Virol.* **35**, 573–577.

Emödi, G. (1974). *Acta Paediat. scand.* **63**, 183–187.
Emond, R. T. C., Evans, B., Bowen, E. T. W. and Lloyd, G. (1977). *Br. med. J.* **2**, 541–544.
Engleman, E. G., Sonnenfeld, G., Dauphinee, M., Greenspan, J. S., Talal, N., McDevitt, H. O. and Merigan, T. C. (1981). *Arthritis Rheum.*, in press.
Fog, T. (1979). *In* "Search for the Cause of Multiple Sclerosis and Other Diseases of the Central Nervous System" (Ed. A. Boeze). First International Symposium of Hertie Foundation in Frankfurt/Main.
Greenberg, H. B., Pollard, R. B., Lutwick, L. I., Gregory, P. B., Robinson, W. S. and Merigan, T. C. (1976). *New Engl. J. Med.* **295**, 517–522.
Greenberg, S., Harmon, M. W., Johnson, P. E. and Couch, R. B. (1978). *Antimicrob. Agents Chemother.* **14**, 596–600.
Gresser, I. and Pattison, I. H. (1968). *J. gen. Virol.* **3**, 295–297.
Gresser, I., Maury, C. and Tovey, M. (1976). *Int. J. Cancer* **17**, 647–651.
Gutterman, J. U., Blumenschein, G. R., Alexanian, R., Yap, H. Y., Buzdar, A. U., Cabanillas, F., Hortobagyi, G. N., Hersh, E. M., Rasmussen, S. L., Harmon, M., Kramer, M. and Pestka, S. (1980). *Ann. intern. Med.* **93**, 399–406.
Haverkos, H. W., Pazin, G. J., Armstrong, J. A. and Ho, M. (1980). *New Engl. J. Med.* **303**, 699–700.
Hilfenhaus, J., Karges, H. E., Weinmann, E. and Barth, R. (1975). *Infect. Immun.* **2**, 1156–1158.
Hill, N. O., Pardue, A., Khan, A., Aleman, C., Dorn, G. and Hill, J. M. (1981). *J. clin. Hemat. Oncol.* **2**, 23–35.
Hooks, J. J., Moutsopoulos, H. M., Geis, S. A., Stahl, N. I., Decker, J. L., Notkins, A. (1979). *New Engl. J. Med.* **301**, (1), 5–8.
Huddlestone, J. R. and Oldstone, M. B. A. (1979). *J. Immun.* **123**, 1615–1618.
Imanishi, J., Karaki, T., Sasaki, O., Matsuo, A., Oishi, K., Pak, C. B., Kishida, T., Toda, S. and Nagata, H. (1980). *J. Interferon Res.* **1**, 169–179.
Jones, B. R., Galbraith, J. E. K. and Al-Hussaini, M. K. (1962). *Lancet* **i**, 875–879.
Jordan, G. W., Fried, R. P. and Merigan, T. C. (1974). *J. infect. Dis.* **130**, 56–62.
Kajander, A., Essen, R., Isomaki, H. and Cantell, K. (1979). *Lancet* **i**, 984–985.
Kovanen, J., Haltia, M. and Cantell, K. (1980). *Br. med. J.* **280**, 902.
Krown, S. C., Stoopler, M. D., Cunningham, R. S., Oettgen III, S. (1980). *Proc. Am. Ass. Cancer Res.* Abstr. 715.
Langford, M. P., Yin-Murphy, M., Ho, Y. M., Barber, J. C., Baron, S. and Stanton, G. J. (1980). *Infect. Immun.* **29**, 995–998.
Larsson, A., Forsgren, M., Hard af Segerstad, S., Strander, H. and Cantell, K. (1976). *Acta Paediatr. scand.* **65**, 105–110.
Mellstedt, H., Bjorkholm, M., Joannoson, B., Ahre, A., Holm, G. and Strander, H. (1979). *Lancet* **ii**, 245–247.
Merigan, T. C. (1967). *Am. J. Med.* **43**, 817–821.
Merigan, T. C. (1980). *J. infect. Dis.* **141**, 265–270.
Merigan, T. C., Reed, S. E., Hall, T. S. and Tyrrell, D. A. J. (1973). *Lancet* **i**, 563–567.
Merigan, T. C., Rand, K. H., Pollard, R. B., Abdallah, P. S., Jordan, G. W. and Fried, R. P. (1978a). *New Engl. J. Med.* **298**, 981–987.
Merigan, T. C., Sikora, K., Breeden, J. H., Levy, R. and Rosenberg, S. A. (1978b). *New Engl. J. Med.* **299**, 1449–1453.
Merigan, T. C., Gallagher, J. G., Pollard, R. B. and Arvin, A. M. (1981). Antimicrob. Agents Chemother. **19**, 193–195.
O'Reilly, R. J., Everson, L. K., Emödi, G., Hansen, J., Smithwick, E. M.,

Grimes, E., Pahwa, S., Pahwa, R., Schwartz, S., Armstrong, D., Siegel, F. P., Gupta, S., Dupont, B. and Good, R. A. (1976). *Clin. Immun. Immunopath.* **6**, 51–61.

Osther, K., Salford, L. G., Hornmark-Stenstam, B., Flodgren, P., Christophersen, I. S., Magnusson, K. The Southern Sweden Neuro Oncology Group. (1981). *In* "The Biology of the Interferon System." Elsevier/North-Holland Biomedical Press, New York.

Patterson, A., Fox, A. D., Davies, G., Maguire, C. H., Sellors, P. J., Wright, P., Rice, N. S. C., Cobb, B. and Jones, B. R. (1963). *Opthal. Soc. U.K.* **83**, 583–591.

Pazin, G. J., Armstrong, J. A., Lam, M. T., Tarr, G. C., Jannetta, P. J. and Ho, M. (1979). *New Engl. J. Med.* **301**, 225–230.

Pollard, R. B., Egbert, P. R., Gallagher, J. G. and Merigan, T. C. (1980). *Ann. intern. Med.* **93**, 655–664.

Priestman, T. J. (1980). *Lancet* **ii**, 113–118.

Rand, K. H., Rosenbloom, A. L., Maelaren, N. K., Silverstein, J. H., Riley, W. J., Butterworth, B., Yoon, J. K., Rubenstein, A. H. and Merigan, T. C. (1981). *Diabetologia*, **243**, 116–119.

Romano, A., Revel, M., Guarari-Rotman, D., Blumenthal, M. and Stein, R. (1980). *J. Interferon Res.* **1**, 95–100.

Rossi, G. B., Matarese, G. P. and Grappelli, C. (1977). *Nature, Lond.* **267**, 50–52.

Sacks, S. L., Scullard, G. H., Pollard, R. B., Gregory, P. B., Robinson, W. S. and Merigan, T. C. (1981). *Antimicrob. Agents Chemother.*, in press.

Salmon, S. E., Hamburger, A. W., Soehnlen, B., Durie, B. C., Alberts, D. S. and Moon, T. E. (1978). *New Engl. J. Med.* **293**, 1321–1327.

Scott, G. M. and Csonka, G. W. (1979). *Br. J. vener. Dis.* **55**, 442–445.

Scott, G. M. and Tyrrell, D. A. J. (1980). *Br. med. J.* **280**, 1558–1562.

Scullard, G. H., Alberti, A., Wansbrough-Jones, M. H., Howard, C. R., Eddelston, A. L., Zuckerman, A. J., Cantell, K. and Williams, R. (1978). *J. clin. lab. Immun.* **1**, 277–288.

Scullard, G. H., Greenberg, H. B., Smith, J. L., Gregory, P. B., Merigan, T. C. and Robinson, W. S. (1981a). *Hepatology*, in press.

Scullard, G. H., Ljudevit, L. A., Greenberg, H. B., Smith, J. L., Sawhney, V. K., Neal, E. A., Mahal, A. S., Popper, H., Merigan, T. C., Robinson, W. S. and Gregory, P. B. (1981b). *Hepatology,* **1**, 228–232.

Scullard, G. H., Pollard, R. B., Smith, J. L., Sacks, S. L., Gregory, P. B., Robinson, W. S. and Merigan, T. C. (1981c). *J. infect. Dis.,* **143**, 772–783.

Soloviev, V. D. (1969). *Bull. Wld Hlth Org.* **41**, 683–690.

Sonnenfeld, G., Mandel, A. D. and Merigan, T. C. (1978). *Cell. Immun.* **40**, 285–293.

Stanton, G. J., Langford, M. P. and Baron, S. (1977). *Immunology* **18**, 370–376.

Stevens, D. A. and Merigan, T. C. (1972). *J. clin. Invest.* **51**, 1170–1178.

Stewart II, W. E. (1979). *In* "The Interferon System". Springer-Verlag, Vienna, New York.

Strander, H. (1977). *Blut* **35**, 277–288.'

Sullivan, J. L., Byron, K. S., Brewster, F. E. and Purtilo, D. T. (1980). *Science, N.Y.* **210**, 543–545.

Sundmacher, R., Cantell, K., Skoda, R., Hallermann, C. and Newuann-Haefelin, D. (1978). *Albrecht von Graefes Arch. klin. Ophthalmol.* **208**, 229–233.

Taylor, W. F., Irvins, J. C., Dahlin, J. C., Edmonson, J. H., Pritchard, D. J. (1978). *Mayo Clinic Proc.* **53**, 695–700.

Treuner, J. *et al.* (1980). *Lancet* **i**, 817–818.
Vallbracht, A., Treuner, J., Flehmig, B., Josester, K. E. and Niethamer, D. (1981). *Nature, Lond.* **289**, 496–497.
Vantrappen, G., Coremans, G., Billiau, A. and De Somer, P. (1980). Yugoslav Academy of Sciences and Arts. In press.
Virelizier, J. L., Lenoir, G. and Griscelli, G. (1978). *Lancet* **ii**, 231.
Weimar, W., Heijtink, R. A., Schalm, S. W. *et al.* (1977). *Lancet* **ii**, 1282.
Weimar, W., Schellekens, H. and Lameijer, L. D. F. *et al.* (1978). *Eur. J. clin. Invest.* **8**, 255-258.
Weimar, W., Heijtink, R. A., Schalm, S. W. and Schellekens, H. (1979). *Eur. J. clin. Invest.* **9**, 151–154.
Weimar, W., Ten Cate, F. J. P., Masurel, N., Heijtink, R. A., Schalm, S. W. and Schellekens, H. (1980). *Lancet* **i**, 336–338.
Zeng, Y., Liu, G., Chen, S., Wei, J., Zhu, J. and Zai, H. (1979). *Chinese J. Oncology* **1**, 2–7.

INTERFERON

Number 3 in this highly acclaimed series continues the style and format of the previous volumes. It contains seven contributions by internationally recognized authorities covering such areas as interferon's place within the immune system, the production of interferon and a discussion of the present possibilities of, and future hopes for, the clinical use of human interferons.

From the reviews of volume 1

"This book represents something of a new concept in review writing. It is neither a research journal nor an annual publication to summarise the field comprehensively. Rather, it comprises a collection of papers by six different authors, well known for their particular fields, who present their personal views on specific aspects of research into the biology and clinical potential of the interferons. It is the first of what is intended to become a series of such "state of the art" surveys on interferon. Subsequent volumes are promised at approximately yearly intervals. This approach is highly commendable in that it brings together new material from widely different areas of activity, which will be of interest to virologists, immunologists, biochemists and clinical and experimental oncologists . . . In summary, the publishers are to be congratulated on the rapid production of a comparatively cheap collection of pertinent reviews . . . Future volumes in this series will be awaited with interest."

Michael Clemens in **The Journal of Medical Microbiology**

INTERFERON 1 1979

Editor-in-chief: Ion Gresser
1979, xii + 164pp.
0.12.302250.9

Contents

Kari Cantell: Why is interferon not in clinical use today? *William E. Stewart II:* Varied biologic effects of interferon. *Robert M. Friedman:* Interferons: interactions with cell surfaces. *Edward De Maeyer and Jacqueline De Maeyer-Guignard:* Considerations on mouse genes influencing interferon production and action. *Michel Revel:* Molecular mechanisms involved in the antiviral effects of interferon.

INTERFERON 2 1980

Editor-in-chief: Ion Gresser
1980, xii + 100pp
0.12.302251.7

Contents

Ernest K. Knight, Jr: Purification and characterization of interferons. *Joyce Taylor-Papadimitriou:* Effects of interferons on cell growth and function. *Derek C. Burke:* The type I human interferon gene system; chromosomal location and control of gene expression. *N.B. Finter and K.H. Fantes:* The purity and safety of interferons prepared for clinical use: the case for lymphoblastoid interferon. *Stanley Cohen and Pierluigi E. Bigazzi:* Lymphokines, cytokines and interferon(s). Interferon Nomenclature: report from the Committee on Interferon Nomenclature.

ACADEMIC PRESS

A Subsidiary of Harcourt Brace Jovanovich, Publishers
London New York Toronto Sydney San Francisco

Academic Press, Inc. (London) Ltd: 24-28 Oval Road, London NW1 7DX, England
Academic Press, Inc: 111 Fifth Avenue, New York, NY 10003, USA
Academic Press Canada: 55 Barber Greene Road, Don Mills, Ontario M3C 2A1, Canada
Academic Press Australia: Post Office Box 300, North Ryde, NSW 2113, Australia
Academic Press, Japan, Inc: Iidabashi Hokoku Bldg, 3-11-13, Iidabashi, Chiyoda-ku, Tokyo 102, Japan
Academic Press do Brasil Editora Ltda: Praca Jorge de Lima 14, 05503 Sao Paulo, SP, Brazil
Academic Press France: 19-21 Rue de l'Ancienne Comedie, 75006 Paris, France

Printed in England

0.12.302252.5